DASH DIET

Discovering wellness with dash diet

TABLE OF CONTENTS

© Copyright 2024 - All rights reserved.

Legal Notice:

Disclaimer Notice:

Please note the information contained within this document is for educational and entertainment purposes only. All effort has been executed to present accurate, upto-date, and reliable, complete information. warranties of any kind are declared or implied. Readers acknowledge that the author is not engaging in the rendering of legal, financial, medical, or professional advice. The content within this book has been derived from various sources. Please consult a licensed professional before attempting any techniques outlined in this book. By reading this document, the reader agrees that under no circumstances is the author responsible for any losses, direct or indirect, which are incurred as a result of the use of the information contained within this document, including, but not limited to, — errors, omissions, or inaccuracies.

YOUR OPINION MATTERS

Welcome, dear reader! As you embark on this journey, your thoughts and opinions matter to me. If you find value in this book, I kindly ask you to consider leaving a review on Amazon once you've finished reading. Your insights will not only help other readers discover this book, but also guide me in enhancing my future works. Thank you for your support!

Nathan

INTRODUCTION

The Dietary Approaches to Stop Hypertension, commonly known as the DASH diet, has emerged as a prominent and effective dietary approach for promoting overall health and preventing hypertension. Developed by the National Heart, Lung, and Blood Institute (NHLBI), the DASH diet emphasizes a balanced and nutrient-rich eating plan specifically designed to manage blood pressure and reduce the risk of cardiovascular diseases.

The fundamental principle behind the DASH diet is to encourage individuals to adopt a lifestyle that prioritizes wholesome, nutrient-dense foods while limiting the intake of sodium and other potentially harmful elements. It is not merely a temporary solution but rather a sustainable dietary pattern that promotes long-term well-being.

One of the key elements of the DASH diet is its emphasis on consuming a variety of fruits and vegetables. These foods are rich in essential vitamins, minerals, and antioxidants that contribute to overall health. The diet also incorporates whole grains, lean proteins, and low-fat dairy products, ensuring a well-rounded and nourishing intake of nutrients. The DASH diet places a strong emphasis on reducing sodium intake, a critical factor in managing blood pressure.

By minimizing the consumption of high-sodium foods, such as processed and packaged items, individuals following the DASH diet can help control their blood pressure levels and reduce the risk of hypertension-related complications.

Another noteworthy aspect of the DASH diet is its flexibility. The plan can be adapted to various dietary preferences and lifestyles, making it accessible to a wide range of individuals. Whether someone is a vegetarian, vegan, or has specific cultural or culinary preferences, the DASH diet provides guidelines that can be customized to suit different needs while still promoting cardiovascular health.

The positive impact of the DASH diet on health outcomes. Numerous studies have shown that adopting this eating plan can lead to lower blood pressure levels, improved cholesterol profiles, and a reduced risk of heart disease. Beyond cardiovascular benefits, the DASH diet has also been associated with weight management and a decreased risk of other chronic conditions, such as type 2 diabetes.

Furthermore, the DASH diet aligns with broader dietary recommendations for a healthy lifestyle. It encourages mindful eating, portion control, and a focus on whole, unprocessed foods. By promoting these principles, the DASH diet addresses not only the physical aspects of health but also fosters a positive relationship with food and a sustainable approach to nutrition.

In conclusion, the DASH diet stands as a holistic and evidence-based approach to promoting cardiovascular health and overall well-being. Its emphasis on nutrient-rich foods, moderation, and reduced sodium intake makes it a valuable tool in preventing and managing hypertension. As individuals increasingly prioritize health-conscious choices, the DASH diet offers a practical and flexible framework for cultivating lasting habits that support a healthier, more vibrant life.

CHAPTER 1
What is a dash diet?

The DASH diet, or Dietary Approaches to Stop Hypertension, is a dietary plan designed to help prevent and manage hypertension (high blood pressure). Developed by the National Heart, Lung, and Blood Institute (NHLBI), the DASH diet emphasizes a balanced and heart-healthy approach to eating. Its primary focus is on incorporating nutrient-rich foods that contribute to overall cardiovascular well-being.

The key components of the DASH diet include a high intake of fruits, vegetables, whole grains, lean proteins, and low-fat dairy products. These elements are chosen for their nutritional density and their ability to provide essential vitamins, minerals, and antioxidants. The diet also encourages limited consumption of sodium, promoting healthier blood pressure levels.

In the ever-evolving landscape of nutritional science, the Dietary Approaches to Stop Hypertension (DASH) diet has emerged as a prominent and evidence-based dietary strategy. Originally formulated with a specific health goal in mind, the DASH diet has transcended its initial purpose and evolved into a versatile and comprehensive approach to overall well-being. In this exploration, we delve into the historical context, scientific motivations, and the primary objectives that led to the creation of the DASH diet.

Historical Context:

The DASH diet had its roots in the early 1990s, a period marked by increasing awareness of the role of diet in health outcomes. During this era, cardiovascular diseases, particularly hypertension, were on the rise, posing significant public health challenges.

The Rise of Hypertension:

Hypertension, or high blood pressure, was identified as a major risk factor for cardiovascular diseases, stroke, and other health complications. As the prevalence of hypertension surged, the medical and scientific communities sought strategies to address this silent but pervasive health issue.

Shift in Dietary Paradigms:

The prevailing dietary recommendations of the time were often centred around reducing total fat intake, with less emphasis on specific nutrients. However, the quality of the diet, particularly the types of fats and the overall nutrient composition, plays a crucial role in cardiovascular health.

This prompted a paradigm shift towards exploring dietary patterns that could directly impact blood pressure regulation.

Scientific Motivations:

The scientific motivations behind the creation of the DASH diet were rooted in a desire to develop a dietary approach that could effectively lower blood pressure and, by extension, reduce the risk of cardiovascular diseases. The intricate interplay between various nutrients and their impact on blood pressure regulation, leading to the formulation of a diet rich in specific key nutrients.

Nutrient Focus:

The DASH diet places a strong emphasis on certain nutrients known to influence blood pressure. Key among these are potassium, calcium, and magnesium. These minerals were selected based on existing evidence that suggested their potential to counteract the hypertensive effects of sodium, a common dietary concern.

Sodium Reduction:

High sodium intake was identified as a significant contributor to elevated blood pressure. The DASH diet, therefore, incorporated a reduction in sodium intake as a critical component. By limiting sodium, the diet aimed to mitigate the vasoconstrictive effects that contribute to hypertension, providing a comprehensive approach to blood pressure management.

Role of Macronutrients:

Beyond individual minerals, the DASH diet considers the role of macronutrients in blood pressure regulation. The diet encourages a balanced intake of protein, healthy fats, and complex carbohydrates, emphasizing the importance of overall dietary quality rather than singular nutrient focus.

Primary Objectives:

The creation of the DASH diet was driven by specific objectives aimed at addressing the burgeoning issue of hypertension and improving overall cardiovascular health. The primary goals can be categorized into several key areas, each reflecting a nuanced understanding of the complex relationship between diet and blood pressure.

Blood Pressure Reduction:

The foremost objective of the DASH diet was to develop a dietary approach capable of effectively lowering blood pressure. The diet's design, with its emphasis on potassium-rich fruits and vegetables, calcium from dairy sources, and magnesium-containing foods, aimed to create a synergistic effect that countered the hypertensive impact of sodium.

Scientific Rigor:

The creators of the DASH diet were committed to a scientific approach to its development. The diet underwent rigorous testing through clinical trials, most notably the DASH-Sodium trial. This landmark study provided empirical evidence supporting the effectiveness of the DASH diet in reducing blood pressure and highlighted the nuanced relationship between dietary factors and cardiovascular health.

Feasibility and Adherence:

Recognizing that any dietary intervention's success hinges on its feasibility and long-term adherence, the DASH diet was designed to be practical and inclusive. The creators sought to develop a dietary pattern that could be easily adopted by the general population, minimizing barriers to compliance.

Comprehensive Cardiovascular Benefits:

While blood pressure reduction was the primary focus, the creators of the DASH diet aimed for broader cardiovascular benefits by incorporating nutrient-dense foods with proven effects on lipid profiles and overall heart health. The diet sought to be a holistic approach to cardiovascular disease prevention.

Evolution and Impact:

Since its inception, the DASH diet has undergone continuous refinement and adaptation. While initially designed for hypertension management, its positive effects on various aspects of health have propelled it into the spotlight as a comprehensive and sustainable dietary approach. The diet's evolution reflects the ongoing integration of scientific advancements and a growing recognition of the interconnectedness of diet and health.

Expansion to Other Health Conditions:

Beyond its original focus on hypertension, the DASH diet has demonstrated effectiveness in addressing other health conditions. Its potential benefits in weight management, diabetes prevention, and the reduction of overall cardiovascular risk, showcasing the adaptability and versatility of the dietary principles.

Influence on Dietary Guidelines:

The success and scientific support for the DASH diet have influenced national and international dietary guidelines. Elements of the DASH diet, such as the emphasis on whole, nutrient-dense foods and sodium reduction, have been integrated into broader recommendations for maintaining optimal health.

Public Health Impact:

The DASH diet's impact extends beyond individual health to public health initiatives. As governments and healthcare organizations grapple with the rising burden of chronic diseases, the DASH diet serves as a tangible and evidence-based strategy for promoting cardiovascular health on a population level.

The creation of the DASH diet was a response to a pressing health concern – the escalating prevalence of hypertension and its associated risks. Grounded in scientific inquiry and a nuanced understanding of the relationship between diet and cardiovascular health, the DASH diet has surpassed its original objectives. It has become a versatile and comprehensive dietary approach with implications for a spectrum of health conditions.

The DASH diet's journey from a focused intervention to a widely recognized dietary pattern underscores the dynamic nature of nutritional science. As we navigate an era of increasing chronic diseases and lifestyle-related health challenges, the DASH diet stands as a beacon of evidence-based guidance, offering a blueprint for individuals and healthcare professionals alike. Its legacy lies not only in its impact on blood pressure but also in its ability to inspire a broader conversation about the profound influence of diet on our health and well-being.

CHAPTER 2
Benefits of dash diet

In the quest for optimal health and well-being, individuals often seek dietary patterns that not only satisfy their taste buds but also contribute significantly to their overall health. One such dietary approach gaining widespread recognition is the Dietary Approaches to Stop Hypertension (DASH) diet. Originally designed to lower blood pressure, the DASH diet has evolved into a comprehensive lifestyle choice celebrated for its potential benefits in various aspects of health. This article delves into the extensive range of advantages offered by the DASH diet, encompassing cardiovascular health, weight management, diabetes prevention, and overall promotion of well-being.

Cardiovascular Health:

Blood Pressure Regulation:

The primary raison d'être of the DASH diet is its ability to effectively regulate blood pressure. By emphasizing nutrient-dense foods rich in potassium, calcium, and magnesium, the diet aids in dilating blood vessels and mitigating the effects of sodium, resulting in lower blood pressure levels. Numerous studies have consistently demonstrated the DASH diet's efficacy in reducing hypertension, making it a valuable tool in cardiovascular disease prevention.

Cholesterol Management:

Beyond its impact on blood pressure, the DASH diet has been associated with favourable changes in lipid profiles. The emphasis on whole grains, fruits, and vegetables helps lower LDL (low-density lipoprotein) cholesterol, commonly known as the "bad" cholesterol. Simultaneously, it supports the elevation of HDL (high-density lipoprotein) cholesterol, contributing to an overall improvement in cardiovascular health.

Anti-Inflammatory Properties:

The DASH diet's composition, rich in antioxidants and anti-inflammatory compounds found in fruits, vegetables, and nuts, helps combat chronic inflammation. Chronic inflammation is a known precursor to cardiovascular diseases, and by adopting the DASH diet, individuals may reduce their susceptibility to inflammatory processes that contribute to heart-related issues.

Weight Management:

Promotion of Healthy Eating Patterns:

While the DASH diet was initially designed for blood pressure control, its natural emphasis on whole, nutrient-dense foods aligns with principles conducive to weight management. By promoting the consumption of fruits, vegetables, lean proteins, and whole grains, the DASH diet encourages individuals to adopt sustainable and healthful eating patterns, facilitating weight loss and maintenance.

Balanced Macronutrient Intake:

The DASH diet advocates for a balanced distribution of macronutrients, with an emphasis on lean protein sources, healthy fats, and complex carbohydrates. This balanced approach not only aids in satiety but also prevents extreme fluctuations in blood sugar levels, reducing the likelihood of overeating and promoting weight stability.

Portion Control:

The DASH diet inherently promotes mindful eating by encouraging individuals to focus on portion control. By being cognizant of serving sizes and consuming meals rich in nutrient-dense foods, individuals following the DASH diet may find it easier to manage their caloric intake, contributing to weight control and preventing obesity-related complications.

Diabetes Prevention:

Blood Sugar Regulation:

The DASH diet's emphasis on whole grains and high-fiber foods plays a pivotal role in regulating blood sugar levels. This can be particularly beneficial in preventing and managing type 2 diabetes. The slow release of glucose from complex carbohydrates helps stabilize blood sugar, reducing the risk of insulin resistance and diabetes development.

Improved Insulin Sensitivity:

Adhering to the DASH diet may improve insulin sensitivity, a key factor in diabetes prevention. The diet's composition, rich in fruits, vegetables, and low-fat dairy, contributes to enhanced glucose metabolism, reducing the burden on the pancreas and potentially lowering the risk of developing diabetes.

Overall Well-Being:

Nutrient Density and Micronutrient Intake:

The DASH diet is renowned for its focus on nutrient-dense foods, ensuring that individuals receive a wide array of essential vitamins and minerals. This not only supports cardiovascular and metabolic health but also contributes to overall well-being by addressing potential nutrient deficiencies that can impact various bodily functions.

Cognitive Health:

Emerging evidence suggests a connection between dietary patterns and cognitive function. The DASH diet, with its emphasis on antioxidants and anti-inflammatory foods, may play a role in preserving cognitive health. By reducing oxidative stress and inflammation, the diet may contribute to a lower risk of neurodegenerative conditions, such as Alzheimer's disease.

Reduction of Chronic Disease Risk:

Adopting the DASH diet has been associated with a reduced risk of various chronic diseases, including not only cardiovascular diseases but also certain cancers and kidney disease. The diet's emphasis on whole, minimally processed foods contributes to an overall reduction in inflammation and oxidative stress, mitigating the risk of chronic health conditions.

The DASH diet initially devised to combat hypertension, has emerged as a dietary paradigm celebrated for its multifaceted health benefits. From its primary role in blood pressure regulation to its positive impact on weight management, diabetes prevention, and overall well-being, the DASH diet offers a holistic approach to healthful living. As individuals seek sustainable and evidence-based approaches to nutrition, the DASH diet stands out as a versatile and effective tool for promoting long-term health and preventing a myriad of chronic diseases. Embracing the principles of the DASH diet not only fosters cardiovascular health but also sets the stage for a vibrant and resilient life.

Effectiveness of dash diet

The effectiveness of the Dietary Approaches to Stop Hypertension (DASH) diet has been extensively studied and well-documented over the years. Originally developed as a dietary intervention to lower blood pressure, the DASH diet has demonstrated effectiveness not only in blood pressure control but also in various other aspects of health. Let's explore the effectiveness of the DASH diet across different dimensions:

Cardiovascular Health:

The DASH diet's positive impact extends beyond blood pressure control to cardiovascular health. The DASH diet is associated with a lower risk of cardiovascular diseases, including heart attacks and strokes. The emphasis on whole, nutrient-dense foods contributes to favourable changes in lipid profiles, with reductions in LDL cholesterol and improvements in HDL cholesterol levels.

Long-Term Adherence:

The effectiveness of any diet is contingent on long-term adherence. Studies suggest that individuals can successfully adopt and maintain the DASH diet over extended periods. Its flexibility and inclusion of a variety of foods make it more sustainable for individuals to incorporate into their daily lives compared to restrictive or fad diets.

Public Health Impact:

The DASH diet's effectiveness extends to its potential impact on public health. Given its evidence-based approach and positive outcomes, widespread adoption of the DASH diet has the potential to reduce the population's overall risk of cardiovascular diseases, obesity, and related health issues.

In conclusion, the DASH diet has proven to be effective across multiple health dimensions, including blood pressure regulation, cardiovascular health, weight management, and diabetes prevention. Its evidence-based principles make it a valuable tool for promoting long-term health and well-being. However, individual responses may vary, and it is essential for individuals to consult with healthcare professionals or registered dietitians before making significant dietary changes, especially those with pre-existing health conditions.

CHAPTER 3
Dash Diet Food Groups

The Dietary Approaches to Stop Hypertension (DASH) diet is a popular and well-researched eating plan designed to prevent and manage hypertension, also known as high blood pressure. The DASH diet not only emphasizes the importance of reducing sodium intake but also encourages a balanced and nutrient-rich diet. One of the key aspects of the DASH diet is the classification of food into specific groups, each playing a crucial role in promoting overall health and well-being.

1. Vegetables: The Foundation of the DASH Diet

Vegetables take centre stage in the DASH diet and for a good reason. Rich in vitamins, minerals, fibre, and antioxidants, vegetables contribute to heart health and help manage blood pressure. Dark leafy greens, colourful peppers, tomatoes, carrots, and broccoli are examples of nutrient-packed vegetables recommended in the DASH diet. The goal is to incorporate a variety of vegetables into meals, ensuring a diverse range of nutrients.

2. Fruits: Nature's Sweetness and Nutrient Powerhouses

Fruits are another essential component of the DASH diet. Packed with natural sugars, fibre, and a plethora of vitamins, fruits provide a sweet and nutritious alternative to processed snacks. Berries, apples, oranges, and bananas are popular choices. The DASH diet recommends incorporating a variety of fruits to harness the diverse health benefits they offer while also keeping an eye on portion sizes to manage calorie intake.

3. Whole Grains: Fueling the Body with Fiber and Nutrients

Whole grains form a significant part of the DASH diet, offering complex carbohydrates, fibre, and essential nutrients. Brown rice, quinoa, oats, and whole wheat bread are preferred over refined grains. The fibre in whole grains helps regulate blood sugar levels, improve digestion, and contribute to satiety, aiding in weight management—a crucial aspect of hypertension prevention.

4. Lean Proteins: Building Blocks for Health

Protein is vital for building and repairing tissues, and the DASH diet recommends choosing lean protein sources to promote heart health. Examples include poultry, fish, lean meats, tofu, legumes, and nuts. These options provide essential amino acids without the excess saturated fats found in some high-fat protein sources. The DASH diet encourages incorporating a mix of these protein sources into meals to ensure a well-rounded nutrient profile.

5. Dairy or Dairy Alternatives: Calcium for Bone Health

Calcium is essential for maintaining bone health, and dairy or fortified dairy alternatives are key components of the DASH diet. Low-fat or fat-free options like yoghurt and milk provide the necessary calcium without adding excessive saturated fats. Additionally, these foods contribute to overall nutrient intake, including vitamin D, which is crucial for calcium absorption.

6. Nuts, Seeds, and Legumes: Healthy Fats and Plant-Based Proteins

Nuts, seeds, and legumes offer a combination of healthy fats, protein, and essential nutrients. These foods contribute to satiety and can be instrumental in weight management. The DASH diet recommends incorporating these plant-based options into meals and snacks, promoting a diverse and nutrient-rich eating pattern.

7. Fats and Oils: Choosing Wisely for Heart Health

While the DASH diet acknowledges the importance of healthy fats, it also emphasizes moderation. Olive oil, canola oil, and avocado are preferred sources of monounsaturated and polyunsaturated fats. These fats support cardiovascular health while minimizing the intake of saturated and trans fats, commonly found in processed and fried foods.

8. Sweets: Limiting Added Sugars and Desserts

The DASH diet recognizes that indulging in sweets and desserts occasionally is acceptable but encourages moderation. Reducing added sugars is a key element in managing overall calorie intake and supporting heart health. When sweet treats are included, they should be consumed sparingly, and alternatives like fresh fruit can be chosen to satisfy the sweet tooth.

The DASH diet offers a holistic approach to health by combining a balanced mix of nutrient-dense foods while addressing specific dietary factors linked to hypertension. By emphasizing fruits, vegetables, lean proteins, and whole grains, the DASH diet provides a practical and sustainable framework for individuals looking to improve their overall health and reduce their risk of chronic diseases. Incorporating the principles of the DASH diet into one's lifestyle not only promotes physical well-being but also fosters a positive relationship with food, making it a valuable and accessible dietary choice for a wide range of individuals.

The Role of the DASH Diet in Weight Loss

The Dietary Approaches to Stop Hypertension (DASH) diet has gained widespread recognition for its effectiveness in managing blood pressure and promoting overall cardiovascular health. However, beyond its cardiovascular benefits, the DASH diet may also play a significant role in weight loss. This comprehensive analysis aims to explore the components of the DASH diet, its potential mechanisms for weight loss, and the scientific evidence supporting its efficacy in helping individuals achieve and maintain a healthy weight.

Understanding the DASH Diet:

The DASH diet is a dietary plan designed to prevent and manage hypertension, a condition that significantly contributes to cardiovascular diseases. The fundamental principles of the DASH diet revolve around promoting a balanced and nutrient-rich eating pattern. It emphasizes the consumption of whole foods, including fruits, vegetables, lean proteins, whole grains, and low-fat dairy products, while minimizing the intake of sodium, saturated fats, and added sugars.

Key Components of the DASH Diet:

Fruits and Vegetables: The DASH diet encourages a high intake of fruits and vegetables, which are rich in vitamins, minerals, fibre, and antioxidants. These nutrient-dense foods contribute to satiety and can aid in weight loss by providing essential nutrients without excess calories.

Whole Grains: Whole grains, such as brown rice, quinoa, and whole wheat, are integral to the DASH diet. They provide sustained energy, fibre, and a feeling of fullness, promoting weight loss by reducing overall calorie intake.

Lean Proteins: The DASH diet emphasizes lean protein sources, such as poultry, fish, beans, and nuts. Protein is crucial for muscle maintenance and repair, and its inclusion in the diet can help individuals feel fuller for longer, reducing the likelihood of overeating.

Low-Fat Dairy: The DASH diet recommends low-fat dairy products, which are excellent sources of calcium and protein. These components are essential for bone health and can contribute to a balanced diet that supports weight loss.

Limited Sodium: The DASH diet places strict limits on sodium intake, as excessive salt consumption is linked to hypertension. By reducing sodium intake, the diet promotes fluid balance and may contribute to a reduction in water retention and bloating, factors that can affect body weight.

Potential Mechanisms for Weight Loss:

Caloric Restriction: The DASH diet, by emphasizing nutrient-dense foods and limiting the intake of processed and high-calorie foods, naturally encourages caloric restriction. Consuming fewer calories than the body expends is a fundamental principle for weight loss.

Increased Fiber Intake: The high fibre content of the DASH diet, derived from fruits, vegetables, and whole grains, promotes satiety and helps regulate blood sugar levels. This can contribute to reduced overall calorie intake and improved weight management.

Enhanced Nutrient Profile: The DASH diet ensures that individuals receive a broad spectrum of essential nutrients, which can be especially beneficial when trying to lose weight. Adequate nutrient intake supports overall health and can reduce the likelihood of nutrient deficiencies that might trigger unhealthy eating behaviours.

Scientific Evidence Supporting the DASH Diet for Weight Loss:

Clinical Trials: Several clinical trials have investigated the impact of the DASH diet on weight loss. A study published in the American Journal of Clinical Nutrition found that participants who adhered to the DASH diet experienced significant weight loss compared to those on a typical American diet.

Long-Term Weight Maintenance: In addition to short-term weight loss, the DASH diet has demonstrated effectiveness in long-term weight maintenance. The emphasis on sustainable dietary changes makes the DASH diet a viable option for those seeking lasting results.

Comparison with Other Diets: Comparative studies have been conducted to evaluate the effectiveness of the DASH diet in comparison to other popular weight loss diets. The DASH diet may be as effective, if not more so, than other dietary approaches in promoting weight loss.

Challenges and Considerations:

While the DASH diet shows promise in supporting weight loss, it's essential to acknowledge potential challenges and individual variations in response. Factors such as adherence, lifestyle, and personal preferences can influence the success of any dietary plan. Moreover, individual responses to the DASH diet may vary, and it might not be suitable for everyone.

The DASH diet, initially developed to address hypertension, has emerged as a well-rounded dietary approach that extends beyond cardiovascular health to include weight management. Its emphasis on whole, nutrient-dense foods, coupled with restrictions on sodium and processed foods, aligns with key principles of effective weight loss. Scientific evidence supports the DASH diet as a viable and sustainable option for individuals aiming to lose weight and maintain a healthy lifestyle. As with any dietary plan, consultation with healthcare professionals and personalized adjustments based on individual needs is crucial for optimal results.

Tips to maximize your weight loss

Achieving and maintaining weight loss can be a challenging journey, but with the right strategies, individuals can optimize their efforts for success. This comprehensive guide provides practical tips to maximize weight loss, incorporating evidence-based approaches, lifestyle adjustments, and sustainable habits.

Set Realistic Goals:

Establishing realistic and achievable weight loss goals is essential for long-term success. Break down your ultimate goal into smaller, manageable milestones. This approach not only provides a sense of accomplishment but also makes the weight loss journey less overwhelming.

Create a Sustainable Caloric Deficit:

Weight loss fundamentally relies on creating a caloric deficit, where you burn more calories than you consume. However, extreme calorie restriction is not sustainable in the long run. Aim for a moderate caloric deficit by combining a balanced diet with regular physical activity. Consult with a healthcare professional or a registered dietitian to determine a healthy and realistic calorie target for your specific needs.

Prioritize Nutrient-Dense Foods:

Focus on nutrient-dense foods that provide essential vitamins, minerals, and macronutrients without excessive calories. Incorporate a variety of fruits, vegetables, whole grains, lean proteins, and healthy fats into your meals. These foods not only support overall health but also contribute to a feeling of fullness, helping you control your calorie intake.

Practice Mindful Eating:

Mindful eating involves paying full attention to the eating experience, including the taste, texture, and satisfaction derived from food. Avoid distractions such as television or electronic devices while eating, and savour each bite. Mindful eating can lead to better awareness of hunger and fullness cues, preventing overeating.

Stay Hydrated:

Drinking an adequate amount of water is crucial for overall health and can also support weight loss. Sometimes, the body may confuse thirst with hunger, leading to unnecessary calorie consumption. Aim to drink water throughout the day and consider consuming water-rich foods like fruits and vegetables.

Engage in Regular Physical Activity:

Incorporate both cardiovascular exercise and strength training into your routine. Cardiovascular exercises, such as walking, running, or cycling, help burn calories, while strength training builds muscle mass, which can boost metabolism. Aim for at least 150 minutes of moderate-intensity aerobic exercise per week, along with two or more days of strength training.

Get Adequate Sleep:

Sleep plays a crucial role in weight management. Lack of sleep can disrupt hormonal balance, leading to increased hunger and cravings for unhealthy foods. Strive for 7-9 hours of quality sleep per night to support overall well-being and optimize weight loss efforts.

Monitor Portion Sizes:

Be mindful of portion sizes to avoid overeating. Use smaller plates, bowls, and utensils to create the illusion of larger portions. Additionally, listen to your body's hunger and fullness signals, stopping eating when you feel satisfied rather than overly full.

Keep a Food Journal:

Maintain a food journal to track your daily food intake. This practice increases self-awareness, helping you identify patterns, triggers, and areas for improvement. A food journal can also be a valuable tool for healthcare professionals or dietitians to provide personalized guidance.

Manage Stress:

Chronic stress can contribute to weight gain and hinder weight loss efforts. Practice stress management techniques such as deep breathing, meditation, yoga, or engaging in hobbies to promote emotional well-being. Developing healthy coping mechanisms can prevent emotional eating and support overall weight management.

Build a Support System:

Share your weight loss goals with friends, family, or a support group. Having a strong support system can provide motivation, encouragement, and accountability. Share successes, challenges, and experiences with those who understand your journey.

Be Patient and Persistent:

Weight loss is a gradual process that requires patience and persistence. Understand that setbacks may occur, but view them as opportunities to learn and readjust your approach. Celebrate small victories, stay committed to your goals, and focus on adopting sustainable habits for long-term success.

Maximizing weight loss involves a multifaceted approach that encompasses dietary modifications, regular physical activity, and lifestyle adjustments. By setting realistic goals, prioritizing nutrient-dense foods, practising mindful eating, and incorporating a variety of healthy habits, individuals can optimize their weight loss journey. Remember that each person's path is unique, and it's essential to tailor strategies to individual needs and preferences. Consult with healthcare professionals or registered dietitians for personalized guidance and support throughout your weight loss journey.

CHAPTER 5

Tips to Make the Switch to DASH Diet Eating

Start Gradually:

The DASH diet is a lifestyle change, and a gradual approach is often more sustainable. Begin by incorporating one or two DASH diet principles into your daily meals each week. This could involve adding an extra serving of vegetables, choosing whole-grain options, or opting for lean protein sources.

Meal Planning:

Plan your meals in advance to ensure they align with DASH diet principles. Create a weekly menu that includes a variety of fruits, vegetables, whole grains, lean proteins, and low-fat dairy. Having a plan can simplify grocery shopping and preparation, making it easier to stick to your dietary goals.

Experiment with Recipes:

Explore new recipes that incorporate DASH-friendly ingredients. Look for creative ways to prepare fruits, vegetables, whole grains, and lean proteins. Experimenting in the kitchen can make the transition more enjoyable and help you discover delicious and nutritious meals.

Focus on Fruits and Vegetables:

Strive to fill half your plate with fruits and vegetables. Experiment with different varieties, both fresh and cooked, to keep your meals interesting and diverse. Consider trying new fruits and vegetables regularly to expand your palate.

Make Whole Grains a Priority:

Gradually replace refined grains with whole grains in your diet. Choose whole wheat pasta, brown rice, quinoa, and whole-grain bread to increase fibre intake and enhance the nutritional profile of your meals.

Lean Protein Choices:

Opt for lean protein sources in your meals. Experiment with a variety of proteins, including fish, poultry, legumes, and plant-based options like tofu. This variety ensures a balance of nutrients while adding flavorful components to your dishes.

Mindful Eating:

Practice mindful eating by paying attention to your body's hunger and fullness cues. Eat slowly, savour each bite, and avoid distractions during meals. Being present while eating can help prevent overeating and foster a healthier relationship with food.

Reduce Sodium Gradually:

Gradually reduce your sodium intake by cutting back on processed and packaged foods. Experiment with using herbs, spices, vinegar, and other flavorful alternatives to enhance the taste of your meals without relying on excess salt.

Read Food Labels:

Familiarize yourself with reading food labels to identify hidden sources of sodium and added sugars. Choose products with lower sodium content and minimal added sugars to align with DASH diet principles.

Stay Hydrated:

Water is a crucial component of a healthy diet. Stay hydrated by drinking plenty of water throughout the day. Limit the consumption of sugary beverages and high-calorie drinks, as they can contribute to excess calorie intake.

Incorporate Low-Fat Dairy:

Include low-fat or fat-free dairy products in your diet to ensure an adequate intake of calcium and protein. If you have dietary restrictions or preferences, explore alternatives such as almond milk or soy milk.

Explore Plant-Based Proteins:

Experiment with plant-based protein sources such as beans, lentils, tofu, and nuts. These options not only provide essential nutrients but also add variety to your meals. Gradually incorporating more plant-based proteins can be a sustainable approach.

Be Prepared with Healthy Snacks:

Keep healthy snacks readily available to avoid reaching for processed or unhealthy options. Snack on fresh fruits, vegetables with hummus, or a handful of nuts to satisfy hunger between meals.

Seek Professional Guidance:

If needed, consult with a registered dietitian or healthcare professional for personalized guidance. They can provide tailored recommendations based on your individual health needs, ensuring a safe and effective transition to the DASH diet.

Monitor Your Progress:

Keep track of your progress by maintaining a food journal or using mobile apps that track your food intake. Regular monitoring helps you stay accountable and allows for adjustments as needed.

Celebrate Successes:

Acknowledge and celebrate your achievements along the way. Whether it's consistently adhering to DASH diet principles, reaching a weight loss milestone, or adopting a new healthy habit, positive reinforcement enhances motivation and contributes to long-term success.

Making the switch to the DASH diet is a positive step toward improving cardiovascular health and overall well-being. By incorporating practical tips such as gradual changes, meal planning, mindful eating, and creative cooking, individuals can seamlessly transition to the DASH diet. Remember that the journey is unique for each person, and adopting small, consistent changes can lead to significant improvements over time. Embrace the principles of the DASH diet as a long-term lifestyle, and enjoy the positive impact on your health and vitality.

Tips to Lower Your Sodium Intake

Sodium is an essential mineral that plays a crucial role in maintaining various bodily functions, including fluid balance and nerve signalling. However, excessive sodium intake can lead to health problems such as high blood pressure, heart disease, and kidney issues. The recommended daily intake of sodium for most adults is about 2,300 milligrams, but many people consume much more than that. To promote better health, consider implementing the following tips to lower your sodium intake.

1. Read Food Labels

Become a savvy shopper by carefully reading food labels. Pay attention to the sodium content per serving size, and be wary of hidden sources of sodium like monosodium glutamate (MSG), sodium nitrate, and sodium benzoate. Opt for products labelled as "low-sodium" or "sodium-free" whenever possible.

2. Choose Fresh and Whole Foods

Processed and packaged foods often contain high levels of sodium to enhance flavour and preserve shelf life. Opt for fresh fruits, vegetables, lean meats, and whole grains instead. Cooking from scratch allows you to control the amount of salt in your meals.

3. Cook at Home

Preparing meals at home allows you to have complete control over the ingredients and the amount of salt used in your dishes. Experiment with herbs, spices, and other flavourings to enhance taste without relying on excessive salt.

4. Experiment with Herbs and Spices

Explore the world of herbs and spices to add flavour to your meals without relying on salt. Consider using garlic, onion, basil, oregano, thyme, rosemary, and other herbs to create delicious, salt-free dishes.

5. Limit the Use of Salt While Cooking

When cooking, use less salt than the recipe calls for, or omit it altogether. You can always add a pinch of salt at the table if needed, but often, the natural flavours of the ingredients are enough to make the dish tasty.

6. Rinse Canned Foods

Canned vegetables, beans, and other products can be high in sodium due to the canning process. Rinse these foods thoroughly under cold water before using them to reduce their sodium content.

7. Be Mindful of Condiments

Many condiments, such as ketchup, soy sauce, and salad dressings, can be surprisingly high in sodium. Opt for low-sodium or sodium-free versions, and use them sparingly.

8. Choose Low-Sodium Alternatives

Look for low-sodium or sodium-free alternatives to your favourite foods. This includes items like low-sodium broths, canned goods, and snacks. Gradually transition to these alternatives to allow your taste buds to adjust.

9. Be Cautious with Processed Meats

Processed meats like bacon, sausages, and deli meats are often loaded with sodium. Choose fresh, lean meats, and if you can't resist processed options, look for low-sodium varieties.

10. Control Portion Sizes

Even low-sodium foods can contribute to a high sodium intake if consumed in large quantities. Pay attention to portion sizes to keep your overall sodium consumption in check.

11. Limit Restaurant and Takeout Meals

Restaurant and takeout meals tend to be high in sodium. When dining out, ask for dishes to be prepared with less salt, and avoid adding extra salt to the table. Consider preparing meals at home and bringing them to work to resist the temptation of high-sodium fast food.

12. Gradually Reduce Salt

If you're used to a high-sodium diet, abruptly cutting salt may make your food taste bland. Gradually reduce your salt intake to allow your taste buds to adjust, and experiment with alternative seasonings.

13. Stay Hydrated

Drinking plenty of water can help flush excess sodium from your body. Adequate hydration also supports overall health and can be a simple yet effective way to mitigate the effects of high sodium intake.

14. Choose Fresh Fruits as Snacks

Instead of reaching for salty snacks, opt for fresh fruits like apples, oranges, or berries. Not only are they low in sodium, but they also provide essential vitamins and minerals.

15. Educate Yourself on Sodium Content

Familiarize yourself with the sodium content of common foods. Being aware of high-sodium foods allows you to make informed choices and helps you stay within recommended daily limits.

16. Use Lemon and Vinegar

Enhance the flavour of your dishes with lemon juice or vinegar instead of salt. The acidity can add a refreshing and tangy taste without the need for excess sodium.

17. Choose Unsalted Nuts and Seeds

Nuts and seeds are nutritious snacks, but salted varieties can contribute to high sodium intake. Opt for unsalted versions to enjoy the health benefits without the added sodium.

18. Monitor Your Medications

Some medications, particularly antacids and pain relievers, may contain sodium. Consult with your healthcare provider about alternatives or ways to mitigate the sodium content if you are on medication.

19. Plan Your Meals

Planning meals in advance allows you to control ingredients and portion sizes. It also helps you avoid the last-minute temptation of convenience foods that may be high in sodium.

20. Be Patient and Persistent

Reducing sodium intake is a gradual process, and it requires patience and persistence. Celebrate small victories, and don't be discouraged if progress is slow. Over time, your taste buds will adapt, and your overall health will benefit.

Lowering your sodium intake is a proactive step toward promoting better health and preventing various chronic conditions. By making mindful choices, reading labels, and gradually adopting healthier eating habits, you can successfully reduce your sodium intake without sacrificing flavour. Remember that small changes add up, and your body will thank you for prioritizing its well-being. Always consult with a healthcare professional for personalized advice, especially if you have existing health conditions or concerns.

The DASH Diet and Its Impact on Hypertension

The DASH diet, which stands for Dietary Approaches to Stop Hypertension, is a dietary plan designed to help prevent and manage hypertension, or high blood pressure. It emphasizes a balanced and nutrient-rich approach to eating, with a focus on foods that are known to lower blood pressure.

Here are some key features of the DASH diet and its impact on hypertension:

Emphasis on Fruits and Vegetables: The DASH diet encourages the consumption of fruits and vegetables, which are rich in potassium, magnesium, and fibre. These nutrients have been associated with lower blood pressure.

Whole Grains: The diet promotes the consumption of whole grains, such as brown rice, quinoa, and whole wheat bread. Whole grains provide essential nutrients and fibre, contributing to heart health.

Lean Protein Sources: The DASH diet recommends lean protein sources, such as poultry, fish, beans, and nuts, instead of red meat and processed meats. These protein sources are lower in saturated fat, which is beneficial for heart health.

Dairy: Low-fat or fat-free dairy products are encouraged on the DASH diet. These provide calcium and other nutrients without the added saturated fat of full-fat dairy.

Limited Sodium Intake: The DASH diet places a strong emphasis on reducing sodium intake, as high sodium levels can contribute to elevated blood pressure. This involves reducing the consumption of processed and packaged foods, as they often contain high levels of sodium.

Moderate Alcohol Consumption: If individuals choose to drink alcohol, the DASH diet suggests doing so in moderation. For most adults, moderate alcohol consumption is defined as up to one drink per day for women and up to two drinks per day for men.

Following the DASH diet can lead to significant reductions in blood pressure. The diet's focus on nutrient-dense, whole foods and the restriction of sodium intake are believed to contribute to its effectiveness in managing hypertension.

It's important to note that the DASH diet is not a quick-fix solution, and its benefits are best realized when it is adopted as a long-term lifestyle change. Individuals with hypertension or those looking to prevent it should consider consulting with a healthcare professional or a registered dietitian to tailor the DASH diet to their specific needs and medical conditions. Additionally, lifestyle factors such as regular physical activity and weight management also play important roles in blood pressure control.

CHAPTER 6
Recipes for dash diet

Classic Lemon Herb Marinade

Grilled Lemon Herb Chicken is a fantastic and flavorful dish that's perfect for a summer cookout or a quick weeknight meal. Here are the ingredients and instructions for two popular variations:

Option 1: Classic Lemon Herb Marinade

Ingredients:

- 4 boneless, skinless chicken breasts (about 1 pound)
- 1/4 cup olive oil
- 1/4 cup lemon juice
- 2 tablespoons fresh thyme leaves
- 2 tablespoons fresh rosemary leaves, chopped
- 2 cloves garlic, minced
- 1 teaspoon salt
- 1/2 teaspoon black pepper

Instructions:

Combine all marinade ingredients in a bowl or ziplock bag. Add chicken and toss to coat evenly. Marinate for at least 30 minutes or up to 4 hours for deeper flavour.

Preheat the grill to medium-high heat. Oil the grates lightly.
Remove chicken from marinade and discard any excess.
Grill chicken for 5-7 minutes per side or until cooked
through (internal temperature reaches 165°F).
Serve immediately with grilled lemon wedges and your
favourite sides.

Option 2: Mediterranean-inspired Herb Marinade
Ingredients:

- 4 boneless, skinless chicken breasts (about 1 pound)
- 1/4 cup olive oil
- 1/4 cup chopped fresh parsley
- 2 tablespoons chopped fresh mint
- 2 tablespoons chopped fresh oregano
- 2 tablespoons lemon zest
- 1 teaspoon dried thyme
- 1/2 teaspoon salt
- 1/4 teaspoon black pepper

Instructions:

• Follow steps 1-3 from Option 1, using the Mediterranean-inspired marinade ingredients.

• Serve with crumbled feta cheese, chopped Kalamata olives, and a drizzle of lemon juice.

Tips:

For extra char and flavour, place lemon slices directly on the grill alongside the chicken during the last few minutes of cooking.

If your chicken breasts are uneven in thickness, pound them gently with a meat mallet to create a more even cooking surface.

Chicken is done when it reaches an internal temperature of 165°F. Check the temperature with a meat thermometer inserted into the thickest part of the chicken breast.

Let the chicken rest for 5-10 minutes before slicing to allow the juices to redistribute, resulting in juicier meat.

No matter which variation you choose, Grilled Lemon Herb Chicken is sure to be a crowd-pleaser. Enjoy!

Quinoa Salad with Veggies

Quinoa salad with veggies is a fantastic choice for a light and refreshing lunch, a hearty side dish, or even a picnic! Here's what you'll need to get started:

Ingredients:

Quinoa: 1 cup uncooked quinoa (yields approximately 3 cups cooked)

Vegetables: Choose 3-4 of your favorites! Some good options include:

- Bell peppers (red, yellow, orange) - chopped
- Cucumber - diced
- Cherry tomatoes - halved
- Carrots - shredded
- Zucchini - spiralized or chopped
- Broccoli florets - steamed or roasted
- Edamame - shelled
- Corn kernels - fresh or frozen
- Red onion - thinly sliced (optional)
- Fresh herbs: Chopped parsley, cilantro, mint, or basil (optional)
- Dressing: This is where you can get creative! Here are a few ideas:
- Lemon vinaigrette: Whisk together olive oil, lemon juice, Dijon mustard, salt, and pepper.
- Balsamic vinaigrette: Combine balsamic vinegar, olive oil, honey, salt, and pepper.
- Creamy herb dressing: Blend fresh herbs like parsley, cilantro, or mint with plain yoghurt, olive oil, lemon juice, garlic, and salt.

Instructions:

• Cook the quinoa: Rinse the quinoa in a fine-mesh strainer. In a saucepan, combine quinoa with water or broth (according to package instructions). Bring to a boil, then reduce heat and simmer for 15-20 minutes or until cooked through and fluffy. Fluff with a fork and set aside to cool slightly.

• Prepare the vegetables: Wash and chop your chosen veggies. If using raw vegetables, ensure they are finely chopped for optimal texture.

• Combine everything: In a large bowl, combine the cooled quinoa, vegetables, and fresh herbs (if using).

• Dress to impress: Drizzle your chosen dressing over the salad and gently toss to coat everything evenly. Taste and adjust seasoning as needed.

Tips:

For added protein, toss in cooked chickpeas, lentils, or grilled chicken/fish.

Roasted vegetables can add a deeper flavour. Simply toss your chosen veggies with olive oil, salt, and pepper, then roast at 400°F for 15-20 minutes until tender.

Leftovers can be stored in an airtight container in the fridge for up to 3 days.

Baked Salmon with Dill

Aked salmon with dill is a classic dish that's easy to prepare and delivers amazing flavour. Here are two delicious options for you:

Option 1: Simple and herb-y

Ingredients:

- 4 salmon fillets (around 5-6 oz each)
- 2 tablespoons olive oil
- 1 1/2 tablespoons fresh dill, chopped
- 1 teaspoon lemon juice
- 1/2 teaspoon salt
- 1/4 teaspoon black pepper

Instructions:

• Preheat your oven to 400°F (200°C). Line a baking sheet with parchment paper.

• In a small bowl, whisk together olive oil, dill, lemon juice, salt, and pepper.

• Brush the salmon fillets generously with the herb mixture on both sides.

• Place the salmon on the prepared baking sheet and bake for 12-15 minutes, or until cooked through and flakes easily with a fork.

• Serve immediately with your favourite sides, like roasted vegetables, rice, or a salad.

Option 2: Lemon Dill Sauce

Ingredients:

- 4 salmon fillets (around 5-6 oz each)
- 1/4 cup plain Greek yogurt

- 1/4 cup mayonnaise
- 1 tablespoon fresh dill, chopped
- 1 tablespoon lemon juice
- 1 teaspoon Dijon mustard
- 1/2 teaspoon garlic powder
- 1/4 teaspoon salt
- 1/4 teaspoon black pepper

Instructions:

• Preheat your oven to 400°F (200°C). Line a baking sheet with parchment paper.

• In a small bowl, whisk together all sauce ingredients.

• Place salmon fillets on the prepared baking sheet and season with salt and pepper.

• Spread the lemon dill sauce evenly over the top of the salmon.

• Bake for 15-20 minutes, or until salmon is cooked through and flakes easily with a fork.

• Serve immediately with your favourite sides, like roasted potatoes or lemon rice.

Tips:

For extra flavour, you can add a thin layer of thinly sliced lemon or onion under the salmon before baking.

If you prefer a crispy skin, broil the salmon for the last 2-3 minutes of cooking.

To check if the salmon is cooked, insert a fork into the thickest part. It should flake easily.

Vegetable Stir-Fry

A vegetable stir-fry is a fantastic way to whip up a healthy and flavorful meal in no time. The beauty lies in its flexibility - you can use any seasonal vegetables you have on hand and personalize them to your taste. Here's a basic guide to get you started:

Ingredients:

- Vegetables: Choose at least 3-4 of your favorites! Some great options include:
- Bell peppers (red, yellow, orange) - sliced
- Broccoli florets
- Snap peas
- Carrots - julienned
- Zucchini - sliced
- Green beans - trimmed and halved
- Mushrooms - sliced
- Spinach or kale - roughly chopped
- Protein (optional): Tofu, tempeh, chickpeas, lentils, or thinly sliced chicken/shrimp
- Aromatics:
- 1-2 cloves garlic, minced
- 1 inch fresh ginger, grated

- Cooking Oil: Neutral oil like peanut, canola, or vegetable oil
- Sauce: This is where you can get creative! Here are a few ideas:
- Simple Stir-Fry Sauce: Soy sauce, rice vinegar, honey, sesame oil, cornstarch
- Spicy Peanut Sauce: Peanut butter, soy sauce, sriracha, lime juice, honey
- Ginger Garlic Sauce: Soy sauce, rice vinegar, honey, ginger, garlic

Instructions:

• Prep your vegetables: Wash and chop all your chosen vegetables into similar sizes for even cooking. If using protein, marinate or season it beforehand.

• Heat your pan: Heat your wok or large skillet over high heat with 1-2 tablespoons of oil.

• Stir-fry the aromatics: Add garlic and ginger, and cook for 30 seconds until fragrant.

• Cook the protein (if using): Add your protein and cook until browned and cooked through.

• Add hard vegetables: Add tougher vegetables like carrots and broccoli, and stir-fry for 2-3 minutes.

• Add softer vegetables: Follow with softer vegetables like mushrooms and bell peppers, and stir-fry for another 1-2 minutes.

• Mix in your sauce: Drizzle in your chosen sauce and toss everything to coat evenly.

• Finish with leafy greens (if using): Add spinach or kale and stir-fry for just 30 seconds until wilted.

• Serve immediately: Enjoy your stir-fry over rice, noodles, or quinoa, garnished with sesame seeds or chopped green onions if desired.

Tips:

For a crispier texture, don't overcrowd the pan and stir-fry in batches if necessary.

Adjust cooking times for vegetables based on their hardness. Don't overcook the vegetables, and they should be tender-crisp for the best flavor and texture.

Feel free to experiment with different sauces and protein options to create your own signature stir-fry!

Mediterranean Chickpea Salad

A Mediterranean chickpea salad is a burst of flavour and freshness, combining protein-packed chickpeas with vibrant vegetables and a tangy vinaigrette. It's perfect for a light lunch, a satisfying side dish, or even a picnic treat!

Ingredients:

- 2 (15-ounce) cans of chickpeas, drained and rinsed

- 1 large cucumber, diced
- 1 red bell pepper, diced
- 2 cups cherry tomatoes, halved
- ¼ cup red onion, diced (optional)
- 4 ounces feta cheese, crumbled
- ¼ cup finely chopped parsley
- Lemon vinaigrette:
- 2 tablespoons olive oil
- 1 tablespoon lemon juice
- 1 teaspoon Dijon mustard
- 1/2 teaspoon dried oregano
- Salt and pepper to taste

Instructions:

• Combine all salad ingredients in a large bowl.

• In a separate small bowl, whisk together the olive oil, lemon juice, Dijon mustard, oregano, salt, and pepper for the vinaigrette.

• Pour the vinaigrette over the salad and toss gently to coat.

• Serve immediately or chill for at least 30 minutes for deeper flavours.

Tips:

For a heartier salad, add cooked quinoa or brown rice.

If you prefer a smoother texture, mash some of the chickpeas with a fork before adding them to the salad.

Get creative with the vegetables! Other great options include Kalamata olives, artichoke hearts, or zucchini.

For a touch of sweetness, add chopped dried fruit like apricots or cranberries.

Leftovers can be stored in an airtight container in the refrigerator for up to 3 days.

Additional Variations:

Spicy: Add a pinch of red pepper flakes or a chopped chili pepper to the vinaigrette.

Creamy: Stir in a spoonful of plain Greek yoghurt to the vinaigrette for a richer flavour.

Herb-forward: Add additional chopped fresh herbs like mint, basil, or dill.

Turkey and Veggie Skewers

Turkey and veggie skewers are a fantastic option for a quick, healthy, and flavorful meal. They're versatile, customizable, and perfect for grilling, baking, or even pan-frying. Here are some ideas to get you started:

Ingredients:

For the Meat:

- Turkey: You can use ground turkey, boneless, skinless turkey breast or thigh, cut into cubes. Around 1 pound/450g of turkey is a good starting point.
- Marinade (optional): Depending on your preference, you can marinate the turkey for added flavour and moisture. Some popular options include:
- Mediterranean: Olive oil, lemon juice, oregano, garlic, rosemary
- Curry: Yogurt, curry powder, turmeric, ginger, cilantro
- BBQ: Honey, brown sugar, soy sauce, Dijon mustard, smoked paprika

For the Veggies:

- Choose a variety of colourful and flavorful vegetables! Some great options include:
- Bell peppers (red, yellow, orange)
- Onion (red, white, or yellow)
- Zucchini
- Cherry tomatoes
- Broccoli florets
- Mushrooms
- Pineapple chunks (for a touch of sweetness)

- Other add-ons:
- Halloumi cheese cubes
- Tofu cubes (marinated)
- Shrimp (skewered and pre-cooked)

Instructions:

• Prepare the turkey: If using ground turkey, simply mix it with your chosen marinade if desired. If using cubed turkey, cut it into uniform pieces and marinate for at least 30 minutes (up to 4 hours) if using.

• Prep the veggies: Wash and chop your chosen vegetables into similar sizes for even cooking.

• Assemble the skewers: Thread the turkey and veggies onto the skewers in an alternating pattern. Aim for a balance of colour and texture.

• Cook the skewers: You have several options:

• Grill: Preheat your grill to medium-high heat. Lightly oil the grates and cook the skewers for 5-7 minutes per side, or until the turkey is cooked through and vegetables are tender-crisp.

• Bake: Preheat your oven to 400°F (200°C). Line a baking sheet with parchment paper and arrange the skewers. Bake for 15-20 minutes, flipping halfway through or until cooked through.

• Pan-fry: Heat a tablespoon of oil in a large skillet over medium heat. Add the skewers and cook for 3-4 minutes per side or until browned and cooked through.

Serving Ideas:

Serve your skewers with rice, quinoa, or couscous.

Add a side salad with a tangy vinaigrette.

Top with tzatziki sauce, hummus, or pesto for extra flavour.

Get creative with dips and sauces to complement your chosen marinades.

Tips:

Soak your wooden skewers for at least 30 minutes before using them to prevent burning.

Brush the skewers with oil before cooking for added browning and flavour.

Don't overcrowd the pan or grill: This can lead to uneven cooking.

Cook until the turkey reaches an internal temperature of 165°F (74°C) for safe consumption.

Feel free to get creative with your ingredients and flavour combinations!

Enjoy your delicious and satisfying turkey and veggie skewers!

Spinach and Feta Stuffed Chicken Breast

Sure, here's a recipe for Spinach and Feta Stuffed Chicken Breasts:

Ingredients

- 4 boneless, skinless chicken breasts
- 1/2 cup chopped fresh spinach
- 1/2 cup crumbled feta cheese
- 1/4 cup chopped red onion
- 2 cloves garlic, minced
- 1/4 teaspoon dried oregano
- Salt and pepper to taste
- 1/4 cup olive oil
- 1/4 cup chicken broth

Instructions

• Preheat oven to 375 degrees F (190 degrees C).

• In a medium bowl, combine spinach, feta cheese, red onion, garlic, oregano, salt, and pepper.

• Butterfly each chicken breast by making a horizontal cut through the middle, not cutting all the way through. Open the chicken breast like a book.

• Spread the spinach and feta mixture evenly over the inside of each chicken breast.

• Fold the chicken breast closed and secure with toothpicks.

• Heat olive oil in a large oven-proof skillet over medium heat. Sear the chicken breasts on both sides until golden brown.

• Pour in the chicken broth and bring to a simmer.

• Transfer the skillet to the oven and bake for 20-25 minutes or until the chicken is cooked through.

• Serve immediately.

Tips

If you don't have fresh spinach, you can use 10 ounces of frozen chopped spinach, thawed and squeezed dry.

You can also add other ingredients to the stuffing, such as sun-dried tomatoes, chopped olives, or cooked rice.

To make the dish ahead of time, prepare the chicken breasts and stuffing, then cover and refrigerate for up to 24 hours. Bake as directed before serving.

Brown Rice and Black Bean Bowl

A brown rice and black bean bowl is a customizable and delicious healthy meal, perfect for lunch, dinner, or even meal prep! Here's a basic recipe and some variations to get you started:

Ingredients:

Base:

- 1 cup cooked brown rice (about 1/2 cup dry)
- 1 cup cooked black beans (about 15 oz canned, drained and rinsed)
- Veggies (choose 2-3):
- Chopped bell peppers (red, yellow, orange)
- Diced tomatoes

- Shredded carrots
- Sliced cucumber
- Roasted zucchini
- Chopped avocado
- Fresh herbs (optional):
- Cilantro
- Parsley
- Lime wedges
- Dressing/Sauce (choose 1):
- Cilantro lime dressing: Lime juice, olive oil, honey, Dijon mustard, cilantro
- Avocado crema: Mashed avocado, lime juice, garlic, chilli flakes
- Spicy black bean sauce: Canned black beans, salsa, spices like cumin, chilli powder
- Balsamic vinaigrette: Balsamic vinegar, olive oil, Dijon mustard, salt, pepper

Instructions:

• Cook the brown rice according to package instructions.

• Heat a pan with a little oil (optional) and sauté your chosen veggies until slightly tender-crisp.

• Assemble your bowl! Start with the rice and black beans, then top with your chosen veggies, herbs, and dressing/sauce.

• Enjoy!

Variations:

• Protein power: Add grilled chicken, fish, tofu, or tempeh for a more filling meal.

• Spice it up: Add chopped jalapeños, sriracha, or chilli flakes to your dressing/sauce.

• Go tropical: Add mango, pineapple, or black beans for a Caribbean twist.

• Mediterranean vibes: Top with crumbled feta cheese, Kalamata olives, and chopped red onion.

• Make it hearty: Add quinoa, corn kernels, or roasted sweet potato cubes for extra texture.

Tips:

Cook extra rice and beans for meal prep lunches or bowls throughout the week.

Get creative with your veggies and toppings! Use what you have on hand or explore new flavours.

Adjust the portion sizes based on your hunger and dietary needs.

Don't be afraid to experiment and find your perfect brown rice and black bean bowl combination!

Shrimp and Asparagus Stir-Fry

Shrimp and asparagus stir-fry is a quick, healthy, and incredibly flavorful dish perfect for any weeknight meal.

Here's a classic recipe with some options to customize it to your taste:

Ingredients:

For the stir-fry:

- 1 pound large shrimp, peeled and deveined
- 1 pound asparagus, trimmed and cut into 2-inch pieces
- 2 cloves garlic, minced
- 1 tablespoon fresh ginger, grated (or 1 teaspoon ground ginger)
- 1/4 cup soy sauce
- 1 tablespoon oyster sauce (optional)
- 1 tablespoon rice vinegar
- 1 tablespoon cornstarch
- 1 tablespoon vegetable oil
- 1/2 teaspoon sesame oil (optional)
- 1/4 cup sliced green onions (for garnish)
- For the marinade (optional):
- 1 tablespoon cornstarch
- 1 tablespoon soy sauce
- 1/2 teaspoon rice vinegar
- 1/4 teaspoon white pepper

Instructions:

• Marinate the shrimp (optional): In a bowl, combine cornstarch, soy sauce, rice vinegar, and white pepper. Add the shrimp and toss to coat. Marinate for 15 minutes to 30 minutes if desired.

• Prepare the sauce: In a small bowl, whisk together soy sauce, oyster sauce (if using), rice vinegar, and cornstarch. Set aside.

• Heat the oil: Heat vegetable oil in a large wok or skillet over high heat. Add the shrimp and stir-fry for 2-3 minutes or until just cooked through. Remove from the pan and set aside.

• Stir-fry the vegetables: Add the garlic and ginger to the pan and cook for 30 seconds until fragrant. Add the asparagus and stir-fry for 2-3 minutes or until tender-crisp.

• Combine and finish: Return the shrimp to the pan and pour in the sauce. Stir-fry for 1-2 minutes until the sauce thickens slightly. Drizzle with sesame oil (if using) and garnish with green onions.

• Serve immediately: Enjoy your shrimp and asparagus stir-fry over rice, noodles, or quinoa.

Tips:

For extra flavour, marinate the shrimp for at least 30 minutes.

Don't overcrowd the pan when stir-frying. Cook the shrimp and vegetables in batches if necessary.

Adjust the amount of chilli flakes or sriracha to your desired level of spiciness.

Feel free to add other vegetables to the stir-fry, such as bell peppers, onions, or broccoli.

Serve with a side of steamed rice or noodles for a complete meal.

Variations:

Lemon Garlic: Substitute lemon juice for rice vinegar and add a teaspoon of honey for a brighter, sweeter flavour.

Spicy Peanut: Add 1 tablespoon peanut butter and 1/2 teaspoon red pepper flakes to the sauce for a creamy, spicy kick.

Sesame Teriyaki: Replace the soy sauce with teriyaki sauce and sprinkle with sesame seeds before serving.

Sweet Potato and Chickpea Curry

Sweet potato and chickpea curry is a vibrant and flavorful dish that's perfect for a cosy meal. The sweetness of the roasted sweet potatoes balances beautifully with the savoury chickpeas and aromatic spices. Here's a recipe to get you started, along with some variations to personalize it:

Ingredients:

For the roasted sweet potatoes:

- 2 large sweet potatoes, peeled and cut into 1-inch cubes
- 1 tablespoon olive oil
- 1/2 teaspoon salt
- 1/4 teaspoon black pepper

For the curry:

- 1 tablespoon vegetable oil
- 1 onion, chopped
- 2 cloves garlic, minced
- 1 tablespoon grated ginger
- 1 teaspoon ground turmeric
- 1 teaspoon ground cumin
- 1/2 teaspoon garam masala
- 1/4 teaspoon chilli powder (optional)
- 1 (14.5 oz) can of diced tomatoes, undrained
- 1 (15 oz) can chickpeas, drained and rinsed
- 1 cup vegetable broth
- 1/4 cup chopped fresh cilantro (optional)

Instructions:

• Preheat oven to 400°F (200°C).

• Prepare the sweet potatoes: Toss the sweet potato cubes with olive oil, salt, and pepper. Spread on a baking sheet in a single layer and roast for 20-25 minutes or until tender and slightly golden brown.

• Heat the oil in a large pot or Dutch oven over medium heat. Add the onion and cook until softened about 5 minutes.

• Add the garlic and ginger and cook for another minute until fragrant.

• Stir in the turmeric, cumin, garam masala, and chilli powder (if using). Cook for 30 seconds to release the aromatics.

• Add the diced tomatoes, chickpeas, and vegetable broth. Bring to a simmer and cook for 10 minutes or until slightly thickened.

• Fold in the roasted sweet potatoes and gently stir to combine. Heat through for another 2-3 minutes.

• Garnish with chopped cilantro (optional) and serve immediately over rice, quinoa, or naan.

Variations:

• Coconut Curry: Add 1 cup of coconut milk along with the vegetable broth for a richer and creamier texture.

• Spicy Madras Curry: Increase the chilli powder to 1/2 teaspoon or add a chopped serrano pepper for a bolder kick.

• Green Curry: Substitute green curry paste for the garam masala and chilli powder for a vibrant and fragrant twist.

• Roasted Vegetables: Add in other roasted vegetables like bell peppers, broccoli, or cauliflower for even more flavour and texture.

• Protein Power: Stir in cooked tofu, grilled chicken, or shrimp for a more substantial meal.

Tips:

Adjust the seasonings to your taste. Feel free to add more salt, pepper, or a squeeze of lemon juice for a brighter flavour.

Leftovers can be stored in an airtight container in the refrigerator for up to 3 days. Reheat gently on the stovetop. Serve with your favourite Indian or Thai side dishes, like raita, papadums, or pickled vegetables.

Grilled Veggie Wrap

A grilled veggie wrap is a fantastic, healthy and delicious option for lunch, a light dinner, or even a picnic treat! The beauty lies in its flexibility - you can use any seasonal vegetables you have on hand and personalize them to your taste. Here's a basic guide to get you started:

Ingredients:

• **Wraps:** Choose 4 whole wheat tortillas or your favourite type of wrap (spinach, gluten-free, etc.).

• **Vegetables:** Pick 3-4 of your favorites! Some good options include:

  • Bell peppers (red, yellow, orange) - sliced
  • Zucchini - sliced

- Onions (red or white) - thinly sliced
- Mushrooms - sliced
- Asparagus - trimmed and cut into spears
- Spinach or kale - roughly chopped
- Cherry tomatoes - halved (optional)
- Spread (optional): Hummus, pesto, guacamole, vegan mayo, or your favourite dip.
- Protein (optional): Grilled chicken, tofu, tempeh, or falafel strips.
- Cheese (optional): Feta, goat cheese, mozzarella, or cheddar cheese crumbles.
- Fresh herbs (optional): Chopped parsley, cilantro, basil, or mint.
- Dressing (optional): Lemon vinaigrette, balsamic vinaigrette, or a simple drizzle of olive oil and balsamic vinegar.

Instructions:

• Preheat your grill or grill pan to medium heat. Lightly oil the grates (if using).

• Prepare your vegetables: Wash and chop all your chosen vegetables into similar sizes for even cooking. If using protein, marinate or season it beforehand.

• Grill the vegetables: Arrange the vegetables on the grill or grill pan and cook for 3-5 minutes per side or until tender-crisp. You can grill different vegetables in batches if needed.

• Warm the wraps: Briefly heat the wraps on the grill or in a dry pan over medium heat for about 30 seconds per side. This makes them more pliable and prevents them from tearing.

• Assemble your wraps: Spread your chosen spread, if using, on one half of each wrap. Layer on the grilled vegetables, protein (if using), cheese (if using), and fresh herbs (if using). You can drizzle with dressing if desired.

• Fold and enjoy! Fold the bottom and top edges of the wrap inward, then roll up snugly. Cut the wrap in half diagonally for easier eating.

Tips:

For extra flavour, marinate your vegetables in olive oil, herbs, and spices before grilling.

Don't overcrowd the grill - cook the vegetables in batches if necessary for even cooking.

Adjust the cooking time for vegetables based on their hardness. Spinach and kale just need a quick wilt, while asparagus and zucchini might need a few minutes longer.

Feel free to get creative with your ingredients and flavour combinations! Try different spreads, cheeses, and proteins to find your favourite combination.

Leftovers can be stored in an airtight container in the refrigerator for up to 3 days.

Additional Variations:

Mediterranean: Spread hummus and top with grilled zucchini, red peppers, onions, olives, and crumbled feta cheese. Drizzle with a lemon vinaigrette.

Spicy Southwest: Spread guacamole and top with grilled mushrooms, bell peppers, corn, black beans, and a sprinkle of taco seasoning. Drizzle with sriracha or hot sauce.

Asian Fusion: Spread peanut sauce and top with grilled asparagus, red onions, carrots, and tofu. Drizzle with a sweet and sour sauce.

Lemon Garlic Tilapia

Lemon garlic tilapia is a classic dish for a reason – it's simple, flavorful, and incredibly versatile. Here are two delicious ways to prepare it:

Baked Lemon Garlic Tilapia:
Ingredients:

- 4 tilapia fillets (around 5-6 oz each)
- 2 tablespoons olive oil
- 1 1/2 tablespoons fresh lemon juice
- 1 teaspoon dried oregano
- 1/2 teaspoon salt
- 1/4 teaspoon black pepper
- 2 cloves garlic, minced
- 1/4 cup chopped fresh parsley (optional)

Instructions:

Preheat your oven to 400°F (200°C). Line a baking sheet with parchment paper.

In a small bowl, whisk together olive oil, lemon juice, oregano, salt, pepper, and garlic.

Brush the tilapia fillets generously with the herb mixture on both sides.

Place the tilapia on the prepared baking sheet and bake for 12-15 minutes, or until cooked through and flakes easily with a fork.

Garnish with chopped parsley (optional) and serve immediately with your favourite sides.

Greek Yogurt Parfait

Greek yoghurt parfaits are a delightful and versatile dessert or snack, perfect for satisfying your sweet tooth while packing in some protein and healthy fats. Here's a basic recipe and some variations to get you started:

Basic Greek Yogurt Parfait:
Ingredients:

- 1 cup plain Greek yoghurt (2% or non-fat)
- 1/4 cup granola (homemade or store-bought)
- 1/4 cup fresh fruit (berries, mango, peaches, etc.)
- 1 tablespoon honey or maple syrup (optional)
- Pinch of cinnamon (optional)

Instructions:

- Layer half of the yoghurt in a bowl or glass.
- Top with half of the granola and fruit.
- Drizzle with honey or maple syrup if using.
- Sprinkle with cinnamon if using.
- Repeat steps 1-4 with the remaining yoghurt, granola, and fruit.
- Serve immediately and enjoy!

Variations:

- Get fruity: Swap out the fruit for different options like pineapple, kiwi, bananas, or a fruit salad mixture.
- Go nuts: Add chopped nuts like almonds, walnuts, or pecans for extra crunch and texture.
- Chocolate delight: Drizzle with dark chocolate sauce or sprinkle with cacao nibs for a decadent touch.
- Spice it up: Add a pinch of ground ginger, cardamom, or nutmeg for a warm and exotic flavour.
- Protein power: Stir in chia seeds, hemp seeds, or protein powder for an extra boost of nutrition.
- Creamy dream: Make the parfait extra smooth by blending the yoghurt with fruit or almond milk before layering.
- Make it ahead: Assemble the parfait in individual jars or containers and refrigerate for up to 24 hours. Perfect for a grab-and-go breakfast or snack.

Tips:

Use chilled yoghurt and fruit for a refreshing treat.

To prevent the granola from getting soggy, layer it between the yoghurt and fruit.

Adjust the sweetness to your preference. You can skip the added sweetener if using naturally sweet fruits.

Get creative and have fun experimenting with different flavour combinations!

Enjoy your delicious and healthy Greek yoghurt parfait!

Egg White Omelet with Spinach and Tomatoes

An egg white omelette with spinach and tomatoes is a fantastic choice for a healthy and flavorful breakfast, brunch, or even a light lunch. Here's a simple recipe and some variations to customize it to your taste:

Ingredients:

- 3 large egg whites
- 1 tablespoon milk or water
- Pinch of salt
- Pinch of black pepper
- 1 tablespoon olive oil
- 1/2 cup chopped spinach
- 1/4 cup chopped tomatoes
- 1/4 cup crumbled feta cheese (optional)

- Fresh herbs (optional): chopped chives, parsley, or basil

Instructions:

- In a bowl, whisk together egg whites, milk, salt, and pepper until frothy.
- Heat olive oil in a medium skillet over medium heat. Swirl the oil to coat the bottom.
- Pour in the egg mixture and let it cook undisturbed for about 30 seconds, until the edges begin to set.
- Sprinkle the spinach and tomatoes evenly over the egg mixture. Cook for another minute or two until the spinach wilts slightly.
- Using a spatula, fold the omelette in half. Let it cook for another minute or two until cooked through to your desired doneness.
- Slide the omelette onto a plate. Top with crumbled feta cheese and fresh herbs (optional).
- Serve immediately and enjoy!

Variations:

- **Veggie power:** Add other chopped vegetables like onions, peppers, mushrooms, or broccoli for more texture and nutrients.
- **Go cheesy:** Swap the feta cheese for shredded cheddar, mozzarella, or Swiss cheese.

- **Spicy kick:** Add a pinch of red pepper flakes or chopped chilli peppers for a touch of heat.
- Herb haven: Get creative with different fresh herbs like dill, oregano, or thyme.
- **Make it meaty:** Stir in cooked chicken, turkey, or ham for a more filling option.
- **Oven finish:** After folding, transfer the omelette to a preheated oven at 350°F (175°C) for 2-3 minutes for a fluffy centre.
- **Mini omelettes:** Make smaller omelettes in a smaller skillet for fun presentations and portion control.

Tips:

Use non-stick cooking spray if desired for easier flipping.

Don't overcook the omelette, as it will continue to cook slightly after you remove it from the heat.

Adjust the cooking time based on your desired level of doneness.

Get creative and have fun with your flavour combinations!

Enjoy your delicious and healthy egg white omelette with spinach and tomatoes!

Cauliflower Rice Stir-Fry

Cauliflower rice stir-fry is a fantastic light and healthy option for a quick and flavorful meal. It's a great way to incorporate more vegetables into your diet while still enjoying the satisfying textures and tastes of a traditional stir-fry. Here's a basic recipe and some variations to get you started:

Ingredients:
Base:

- 1 tablespoon avocado oil or vegetable oil
- 1 onion, diced
- 2 cloves garlic, minced
- 1-inch fresh ginger, grated (optional)
- 12 oz riced cauliflower (fresh or frozen, thawed)
- Protein (optional):
- 1 cup diced chicken, tofu, shrimp, or tempeh (pre-cooked or marinated briefly)

Vegetables:

- Choose 2-3 of your favorites! Some good options include:
- Bell peppers (red, yellow, orange) - sliced
- Zucchini - sliced
- Snap peas
- Broccoli florets
- Carrots - julienned
- Mushrooms - sliced

Sauce:

- 1/4 cup soy sauce

* 1 tablespoon oyster sauce (optional)
* 1 tablespoon rice vinegar
* 1 tablespoon water
* 1 teaspoon cornstarch
* Pinch of sriracha or chilli flakes (optional)
* Garnish (optional):
* Chopped fresh cilantro
* Sesame seeds
* Peanuts

Instructions:

* Heat oil in a large wok or skillet over medium-high heat. Add the onion and cook until softened about 5 minutes.
* Add the garlic and ginger (if using) and cook for another minute until fragrant.
* Add the riced cauliflower and cook, stirring frequently, until tender-crisp, about 5-7 minutes.
* If using protein, add it to the pan and cook until heated through.
* Add the chosen vegetables and cook for another 2-3 minutes or until tender-crisp.
* In a small bowl, whisk together soy sauce, oyster sauce (if using), rice vinegar, water, cornstarch, and sriracha or chilli flakes (if using).
* Pour the sauce into the pan and stir-fry for 1-2 minutes until the sauce thickens slightly.

- Garnish with chopped cilantro, sesame seeds, and peanuts (optional) and serve immediately over rice, noodles, or quinoa.

Variations:

- **Sweet and Spicy:** Add 1 tablespoon of honey or brown sugar to the sauce and a pinch of red pepper flakes.
- **Thai Curry:** Substitute coconut milk for water in the sauce and add 1 tablespoon curry paste.
- **Teriyaki:** Use Teriyaki sauce instead of the mixed sauce.
- **Tropical Twist:** Add pineapple chunks, chopped mango, and a sprinkle of toasted coconut flakes.
- **Korean BBQ:** Marinate the protein in Korean BBQ sauce before adding it to the pan.
- **Rainbow Veggie:** Use a variety of colourful bell peppers, carrots, and broccoli for a vibrant dish.

Tips:

Use a food processor or grater to quickly and easily make your own riced cauliflower.

If using frozen cauliflower rice, thaw it completely before cooking.

Don't overcrowd the pan when stir-frying. Cook the ingredients in batches if necessary.

Adjust the number of chilli flakes or sriracha to your desired level of spiciness.

Feel free to add other vegetables and flavours to customize the stir-fry to your taste.

With a little creativity, cauliflower rice stir-fry can be a delicious and healthy staple in your weeknight dinners! Enjoy!

Caprese Salad

The Caprese salad, a classic Italian dish, is a delightful combination of juicy tomatoes, creamy mozzarella cheese, and fresh basil leaves. Its simplicity allows the natural flavours to shine, making it perfect for a light lunch, appetizer, or even a side dish. Here's a basic recipe and some variations to get you started:

Ingredients:

Essentials:

- 2-3 ripe tomatoes, sliced into thick rounds (choose heirloom tomatoes for extra flavour)
- 1 ball fresh mozzarella cheese, sliced into a similar thickness as tomatoes
- Fresh basil leaves, torn or roughly chopped
- Extra virgin olive oil
- Salt and freshly ground black pepper

Optional Additions:

- Balsamic glaze or reduction (for drizzling)
- Red onion, thinly sliced
- Garlic cloves, thinly sliced (lightly fried or rubbed on the serving plate)
- Fresh oregano or thyme leaves
- Capers

Instructions:

- Arrange the tomato slices on a plate or platter.
- Top each tomato slice with a mozzarella slice.
- Scatter fresh basil leaves over the top.
- Drizzle with olive oil, season with salt and pepper to taste.
- (Optional) Drizzle with balsamic glaze or add any desired additional ingredients.
- Serve immediately and enjoy!

Variations:

- **Rainbow Caprese:** Use different coloured heirloom tomatoes for a vibrant and flavorful twist.
- **Grilled Caprese:** Grill the tomato and/or mozzarella slices for a smoky and caramelized flavour.
- **Peach Caprese:** Substitute ripe peaches for tomatoes for a sweet and summery version.

- **Watermelon Caprese:** Swap tomatoes with watermelon slices for a refreshing twist.
- **Burrata Caprese:** Use burrata cheese instead of mozzarella for a creamier and richer experience.
- **Caprese Skewers**: Thread tomato, mozzarella, and basil onto skewers for a fun and portable option.

Tips:

Use the ripest and juiciest tomatoes you can find for the best flavour.

Let the mozzarella cheese come to room temperature before slicing for a smoother texture.

Tear the basil leaves instead of chopping them for a more rustic and flavorful touch.

Adjust the amount of olive oil, salt, and pepper to your preference.

Get creative and have fun experimenting with different ingredients and flavours!

Enjoy your delicious and refreshing Caprese salad!

Chicken and Vegetable Kebabs

Chicken and vegetable kebabs are a fantastic grilling option, offering endless possibilities for flavour combinations and appealing to all kinds of dietary preferences. Here's a basic recipe and some variations to get your grill sizzling:

Ingredients:

Base:

- 1 lb boneless, skinless chicken breasts or thighs cut into 1-inch cubes
- 1 tablespoon olive oil
- 1/2 teaspoon salt
- 1/4 teaspoon black pepper

Vegetables (choose 3-4):

- Bell peppers (red, yellow, orange) - cut into cubes
- Zucchini - cut into thick slices or half-moons
- Onions (red or white) - cut into wedges
- Cherry tomatoes - whole or halved
- Mushrooms - whole or sliced
- Pineapple chunks (optional)

Marinade (optional):

- 1/4 cup yoghurt (plain or Greek)
- 1 tablespoon lemon juice
- 1 teaspoon each thyme, oregano, and paprika
- 1/2 teaspoon garlic powder
- Pinch of chilli flakes (optional)
- Skewers: Wooden or metal skewers soaked in water for at least 30 minutes to prevent burning.

Instructions:

- Marinate the chicken (optional): In a bowl, combine yoghurt, lemon juice, spices, and garlic powder. Add the chicken cubes and toss to coat. Marinate for at least 30 minutes or overnight for deeper flavour.
- Prepare the vegetables: Wash and chop the chosen vegetables into pieces of similar size to the chicken cubes.
- Assemble the kebabs: Thread the chicken and vegetables onto the soaked skewers, alternating and creating colourful combinations. Leave some space between pieces for even cooking.
- Preheat your grill to medium-high heat. Lightly oil the grates if using wooden skewers.
- Grill the kebabs for 8-10 minutes per side or until the chicken is cooked through and the vegetables are tender-crisp.
- Serve immediately with your favourite dipping sauces: yoghurt sauce, tahini sauce, chimichurri, or even just a squeeze of lemon and olive oil.

Variations:

- **Mediterranean:** Marinate the chicken in lemon juice, garlic, oregano, and olive oil. Thread with red onion, bell peppers, olives, and feta cheese crumbles.

- **Teriyaki:** Marinate in teriyaki sauce and skewer with pineapple chunks, broccoli florets, and red onion.
- **Spicy Chipotle:** Marinate in chipotle adobo sauce and lime juice. Thread with corn, zucchini, red onion, and shrimp.
- **Greek Skewers:** Use chicken thighs and marinate in Greek yogurt, lemon, dill, and garlic. Thread with red onion, cherry tomatoes, Kalamata olives, and artichoke hearts.
- **Tandoori:** Marinate in a tandoori paste with yoghurt and lemon juice. Thread with bell peppers, onion, paneer cubes, and pineapple chunks.

Tips:

Use wooden skewers for a traditional look, but metal skewers are easier to turn and clean.

Soak the skewers in water to prevent burning on the grill.

Don't overcrowd the kebabs on the grill for even cooking.

Adjust the cooking time depending on the size of your chicken cubes and vegetables.

Get creative with your marinade and vegetable combinations!

Enjoy your delicious and flavorful grilled chicken and vegetable kebabs!

Quinoa-Stuffed Bell Peppers

Quinoa-stuffed bell peppers are a fantastic vegetarian dish that's bursting with flavour, colour, and nutrition. They're perfect for a satisfying lunch, dinner, or even as a party appetizer. Here's a basic recipe and some variations to get you started:

Ingredients:

For the filling:

- 1 cup quinoa, cooked according to package instructions
- 1 tablespoon olive oil
- 1 onion, chopped
- 2 cloves garlic, minced
- 1/2 cup chopped sweet pepper (any colour)
- 1/2 cup chopped zucchini
- 1 (14.5 oz) can of diced tomatoes, undrained
- 1/2 cup black beans, rinsed and drained
- 1/4 cup chopped fresh cilantro
- 1 teaspoon ground cumin
- 1/2 teaspoon chilli powder (optional)
- Salt and black pepper to taste

For the bell peppers:

- 4 large bell peppers (red, yellow, orange, or a mix)
- Olive oil for brushing

Instructions:

- Preheat oven to 375°F (190°C).
- Prepare the filling: Heat olive oil in a large skillet over medium heat. Add onion and cook until softened about 5 minutes.
- Add garlic and cook for another minute until fragrant.
- Add sweet pepper, zucchini, and tomatoes. Simmer for 10 minutes, stirring occasionally.
- Stir in cooked quinoa, black beans, cilantro, cumin, chilli powder (if using), salt, and pepper. Cook for another 5 minutes or until heated through.
- Prepare the bell peppers: Cut off the tops of the bell peppers and remove the seeds and membranes.
- Brush the inside of the peppers with olive oil.
- Stuff the peppers with the quinoa mixture. Don't overfill, as the quinoa will expand while cooking.
- Place the stuffed peppers in a baking dish and pour a little water into the bottom of the dish.
- Bake for 30-35 minutes or until the peppers are tender and the filling is heated through.
- Serve immediately and enjoy!

Variations:

- **Spicy kick:** Add a chopped jalapeño pepper to the filling along with the garlic.

- **Mexican Fiesta:** Stir in 1/2 cup of corn and a tablespoon of chopped fresh avocado before stuffing the peppers.
- **Greek Goddess:** Use crumbled feta cheese instead of black beans, and add a tablespoon of chopped fresh parsley to the filling.
- **Indian Curry:** Replace the cumin with garam masala and curry powder for an Indian-inspired twist.
- **Mushrooms and Swiss:** Use chopped mushrooms instead of zucchini, and top the stuffed peppers with grated Swiss cheese before baking.

Tips:

Choose bell peppers of similar size for even cooking.

Don't pack the quinoa mixture too tightly into the peppers, as it will expand while baking.

Serve the stuffed peppers with your favourite dipping sauces, like guacamole, hummus, or tahini sauce.

Leftovers can be stored in an airtight container in the refrigerator for up to 3 days. Reheat gently in the oven or microwave.

Lentil and Vegetable Soup

A lentil and vegetable soup is a delightful and hearty dish, perfect for a cosy meal or a light yet satisfying lunch. It's packed with protein, fibre, and nutrients, making it a healthy and flavorful choice. Here's a basic recipe and some variations to get you started:

Ingredients:

Soup base:

- 1 tablespoon olive oil
- 1 onion, chopped
- 2 cloves garlic, minced
- 1 cup chopped carrots
- 1 cup chopped celery
- 1/2 cup chopped bell pepper (any colour)
- 8 cups vegetable broth
- 1 cup dry lentils, rinsed
- 1 (14.5 oz) can of diced tomatoes, undrained
- 1 teaspoon dried thyme
- 1/2 teaspoon dried oregano
- Salt and freshly ground black pepper to taste

Optional additions:

- 1 cup chopped kale or spinach, added in the last 5 minutes of cooking
- 1/2 cup cooked pasta or rice
- 1/4 cup chopped fresh parsley or cilantro for garnish
- Lemon wedges for serving
- Crusty bread for dipping

Instructions:

- Heat olive oil in a large pot or Dutch oven over medium heat. Add onion and cook until softened about 5 minutes.
- Add garlic, carrots, celery, and bell pepper. Cook for another 5 minutes, stirring occasionally.
- Add vegetable broth, lentils, diced tomatoes, thyme, oregano, salt, and pepper. Bring to a boil, then reduce heat and simmer for 20-25 minutes or until the lentils are tender.
- In the last 5 minutes of cooking, stir in the kale or spinach (if using).
- Taste and adjust seasonings as needed.
- Ladle the soup into bowls and garnish with your desired toppings (fresh herbs, lemon wedges, etc.). Serve with crusty bread for dipping.

Variations:

- **Creamy Lentil Soup**: Add 1 cup of coconut milk or heavy cream to the pot along with the broth for a richer texture.
- **Spicy Lentil Soup:** Add a chopped jalapeño pepper or a pinch of red pepper flakes for a kick.
- Italian Lentil Soup: Add a tablespoon of chopped fresh basil and a sprinkle of Parmesan cheese before serving.

- **Moroccan Lentil Soup:** Add a teaspoon of ground cumin, coriander, and turmeric for a Moroccan-inspired flavour.
- **Roasted Vegetable Lentil Soup:** Roast the chopped carrots, celery, and bell peppers in the oven before adding them to the soup for a deeper flavour.

Tips:

Use brown lentils for a nuttier flavour and a slightly longer cooking time.

Don't overcook the lentils, as they will turn mushy.

Adjust the amount of vegetables and broth to your desired consistency.

Get creative and have fun experimenting with different flavours and spices!

With its versatility and adaptability, a lentil and vegetable soup is a dish you can enjoy all year round. So grab your favourite ingredients, get creative, and cook up a pot of this delicious and nutritious soup!

Baked Cod with Herbs

Baked cod with herbs is a fantastically easy and flavorful dish that's perfect for a quick and healthy weeknight meal. The delicate cod pairs beautifully with a variety of herbs, making it adaptable to your taste preferences. Here are two versions with some variations to inspire you:

Lemon Garlic Herb Cod:

Ingredients:

- 4 cod fillets (around 5-6 oz each)
- 2 tablespoons olive oil
- 1/2 lemon, juiced
- 1 tablespoon chopped fresh parsley
- 1 tablespoon chopped fresh dill
- 1/2 teaspoon dried thyme
- 1/4 teaspoon salt
- 1/4 teaspoon black pepper

Optional: Lemon slices and fresh herbs for garnish

Instructions:

- Preheat oven to 400°F (200°C). Line a baking sheet with parchment paper.
- In a small bowl, whisk together olive oil, lemon juice, parsley, dill, thyme, salt, and pepper.
- Brush the cod fillets generously with the herb mixture on both sides.
- Place the cod fillets on the prepared baking sheet.
- Bake for 12-15 minutes or until cooked through and flakes easily with a fork.

- Garnish with lemon slices and fresh herbs (optional), and serve immediately with your favourite sides.

Mediterranean Herb Cod:

Ingredients:

- 4 cod fillets (around 5-6 oz each)
- 2 tablespoons olive oil
- 1 tablespoon chopped fresh oregano
- 1 tablespoon chopped fresh rosemary
- 1/2 teaspoon dried thyme
- 1/4 teaspoon salt
- 1/4 teaspoon black pepper
- 1/4 cup chopped sun-dried tomatoes (optional)
- 1/4 cup crumbled feta cheese (optional)

Instructions:

- Preheat oven to 400°F (200°C). Line a baking sheet with parchment paper.
- In a small bowl, whisk together olive oil, oregano, rosemary, thyme, salt, and pepper.
- Brush the cod fillets generously with the herb mixture on both sides.
- If using, sprinkle the cod fillets with chopped sun-dried tomatoes.
- Place the cod fillets on the prepared baking sheet.

- Bake for 12-15 minutes or until cooked through and flakes easily with a fork.
- Top with crumbled feta cheese (optional) and serve immediately with your favourite sides.

Variations:

- **Spicy kick:** Add a pinch of red pepper flakes or chopped chilli peppers to the herb mixture for a touch of heat.
- **Garlic lover:** Add 1-2 cloves of minced garlic to the herb mixture for extra flavour.
- **Citrus boost:** Drizzle the cooked cod with fresh lemon juice or orange juice before serving.
- **Asian twist:** Use ginger, sesame oil, and soy sauce in the herb mixture for an Asian-inspired flavour.
- **Crispy topping:** Before baking, sprinkle the cod fillets with panko breadcrumbs for a delightful crunch.

Tips:

Use fresh fish for the best flavour.

Don't overcrowd the baking sheet. Cook in batches if necessary.

Adjust the cooking time depending on the thickness of your cod fillets.

Get creative with your herb combinations! There are endless possibilities to explore.

Enjoy your delicious and healthy baked cod with herbs! It's a dish that's sure to become a weeknight staple in your kitchen.

Recipes

Vegetarian Chili

A hearty bowl of vegetarian chilli is a fantastic option for a satisfying and flavorful meal packed with vegetables, protein, and spices. Here are two delicious recipes to get you started, plus some variations to customize it to your preferences:

Black Bean and Sweet Potato Chili:

Ingredients:

- 1 tablespoon olive oil
- 1 onion, chopped
- 2 cloves garlic, minced
- 1 bell pepper (any colour), chopped
- 1 jalapeno pepper (optional, for spice), seeded and chopped
- 1 zucchini, chopped
- 1 sweet potato, peeled and diced
- 1 (15 oz) can black beans, rinsed and drained
- 1 (15 oz) can of kidney beans, rinsed and drained

- 1 (14.5 oz) can of diced tomatoes, undrained
- 4 cups vegetable broth
- 1 tablespoon chilli powder
- 1 teaspoon cumin
- 1/2 teaspoon smoked paprika
- 1/4 teaspoon oregano
- Salt and black pepper to taste

Optional Garnishes: Chopped cilantro, avocado slices, lime wedges, sour cream

Instructions:

Heat olive oil in a large pot or Dutch oven over medium heat. Add onion and cook until softened about 5 minutes.

Add garlic, bell pepper, jalapeno (if using), zucchini, and sweet potato. Cook for another 5 minutes, stirring occasionally.

Add black beans, kidney beans, diced tomatoes with their juices, vegetable broth, chilli powder, cumin, smoked paprika, oregano, salt, and pepper. Bring to a boil, then reduce heat and simmer for 20-25 minutes, or until the vegetables are tender and the chilli has thickened.

Taste and adjust seasonings if needed.

Serve hot with your desired garnishes, and enjoy!

Lentil and Vegetable Chili:

Ingredients:

- 1 tablespoon olive oil
- 1 onion, chopped
- 2 cloves garlic, minced
- 1 carrot, chopped
- 1 celery stalk, chopped
- 1 cup dry green lentils, rinsed
- 1 (14.5 oz) can of diced tomatoes, undrained
- 4 cups vegetable broth
- 1 teaspoon chilli powder
- 1/2 teaspoon cumin
- 1/4 teaspoon smoked paprika
- 1/4 teaspoon dried thyme
- Salt and black pepper to taste
- Optional Garnishes: Chopped fresh parsley, cornbread crumbles, hot sauce

Instructions:

- Heat olive oil in a large pot or Dutch oven over medium heat. Add onion and cook until softened about 5 minutes.
- Add garlic, carrot, and celery. Cook for another 5 minutes, stirring occasionally.
- Add lentils, diced tomatoes with their juices, vegetable broth, chilli powder, cumin, smoked

paprika, thyme, salt, and pepper. Bring to a boil, then reduce heat and simmer for 20-25 minutes, or until the lentils are tender and the chilli has thickened.

- Taste and adjust seasonings if needed.
- Serve hot with your desired garnishes, and enjoy!

Variations:

- **Spicy:** Add a pinch of cayenne pepper or chopped chilli peppers for extra heat.
- **Smoky:** Add a chipotle pepper in adobo sauce for a smoky flavour.
- **Hearty:** Add cooked quinoa or brown rice for a more filling option.
- **Tropical Twist:** Add pineapple chunks and mango for a sweet and fruity twist.
- **Vegan:** Use vegetable broth and omit the cheese or sour cream for a vegan version.

Tips:

Use brown lentils for a heartier texture and additional nutrients.

Don't overcook the lentils, as they will turn mushy.

Adjust the amount of vegetables and broth to your desired consistency.

Get creative and have fun experimenting with different flavours and spices!

Baked Chicken with Rosemary and Garlic

Baked chicken with rosemary and garlic is a timeless classic for a reason – it's simple, flavorful, and perfect for a satisfying weeknight meal. Here's a basic recipe and some variations to inspire you:

Basic Recipe:

Ingredients:

- 4 bone-in, skin-on chicken thighs (around 1-1.5 lbs each)
- 2 tablespoons olive oil
- 2 cloves garlic, minced
- 1-2 sprigs fresh rosemary, chopped (or 1 teaspoon dried)
- 1/2 teaspoon salt
- 1/4 teaspoon black pepper

Instructions:

- Preheat oven to 400°F (200°C). Line a baking sheet with parchment paper.
- Pat the chicken thighs dry with paper towels.

- In a small bowl, whisk together olive oil, garlic, rosemary, salt, and pepper.
- Brush the chicken generously with the herb mixture on both sides.
- Place the chicken thighs on the prepared baking sheet, skin-side up.
- Bake for 40-45 minutes, or until the chicken is cooked through and juices run clear when pierced with a fork.
- Let the chicken rest for 5 minutes before serving.

Variations:

- **Lemon Twist**: Add 1 tablespoon of lemon juice to the herb mixture for a touch of brightness.
- **Honey Glaze:** In the last 10 minutes of baking, brush the chicken with a mixture of 2 tablespoons honey and 1 tablespoon Dijon mustard.
- **Spicy Kick:** Add a pinch of red pepper flakes or chopped chilli peppers to the herb mixture for some heat.
- **Smoky Flavor:** Rub the chicken with smoked paprika before brushing it with the herb mixture.
- **Mediterranean Vibes:** Add chopped sun-dried tomatoes and Kalamata olives to the baking sheet before adding the chicken.

- **Garlic Lover:** Stuff the chicken cavity with additional whole garlic cloves for an intense garlic flavour.

Tips:

Use fresh rosemary for the best flavour. If using dried, add a little more than the recipe suggests.

Don't overcrowd the baking sheet. Cook in batches if necessary.

Adjust the cooking time depending on the size of your chicken thighs.

Get creative with your herb and spice combinations! There are endless possibilities to explore.

Serving suggestions:

Pair your baked chicken with roasted vegetables, mashed potatoes, rice, or couscous.

Add a simple salad and some crusty bread for a complete meal.

Drizzle with pan juices for extra flavour.

Cucumber and Tomato Salad

Ah, the simple yet refreshing cucumber and tomato salad! It's a classic for a reason, offering a beautiful interplay of textures and flavours. Here are some ways to prepare it based on your previous inquiries:

Mediterranean Inspiration:
Ingredients:

- 2 large cucumbers, diced
- 4 Roma tomatoes, diced
- 1/2 red onion, thinly sliced
- 1/4 cup chopped fresh parsley
- 2 tablespoons olive oil
- 1 tablespoon lemon juice
- 1/2 teaspoon salt
- 1/4 teaspoon black pepper
- Pinch of sumac (optional)

Instructions:

- Combine all ingredients in a large bowl.
- Toss gently to coat.
- Let stand for at least 15 minutes to allow the flavours to meld.
- Enjoy!

Quick and Easy:
Ingredients:

- 1 English cucumber, sliced
- 2 large tomatoes, sliced

- 1/2 red onion, thinly sliced
- 2 tablespoons olive oil
- 1 tablespoon red wine vinegar
- 1/2 teaspoon salt
- 1/4 teaspoon black pepper

Instructions:

- Combine all ingredients in a large bowl.
- Toss gently to coat.
- Serve immediately.
- Spicy Kick:

Ingredients:

- 1 cucumber, diced
- 2 tomatoes, diced
- 1/2 red onion, thinly sliced
- 1/4 cup chopped fresh cilantro
- 2 tablespoons olive oil
- 1 tablespoon lime juice
- 1/2 teaspoon salt
- 1/4 teaspoon black pepper
- Pinch of red pepper flakes

Instructions:

- Combine all ingredients in a large bowl.
- Toss gently to coat.

- Serve immediately.

Additional Tips:

For a smoother texture, peel the cucumbers before dicing.

Use ripe tomatoes for the best flavour.

Adjust the amount of onion and herbs to your preference.

Serve the salad on its own, as a side dish, or as a refreshing topping for grilled chicken or fish.

Turkey and Vegetable Skillet

A turkey and vegetable skillet – perfect for a quick, healthy, and flavorful meal!

Mediterranean Vibes:

Ingredients:

- 1 lb ground turkey
- 1 onion, diced
- 2 cloves garlic, minced
- 1 zucchini, diced
- 1 bell pepper (any colour), diced
- 14.5 oz can diced tomatoes, undrained
- 1/2 cup chopped fresh basil
- 1/4 cup chopped fresh oregano
- 1/2 teaspoon dried thyme

- 1/2 cup crumbled feta cheese
- Olive oil
- Salt and pepper

Instructions:

-
- Heat olive oil in a large skillet over medium heat. Brown the ground turkey, breaking it up with a spoon.
- Add onion and garlic, and cook until softened.
- Stir in zucchini and bell pepper, and cook until slightly tender.
- Add diced tomatoes, basil, oregano, thyme, salt, and pepper. Simmer for 10 minutes, allowing the flavours to meld.
- Garnish with crumbled feta cheese before serving.

Spicy Fiesta:

Ingredients:

- 1 lb ground turkey
- 1 onion, diced
- 2 cloves garlic, minced
- 1 can black beans, rinsed and drained
- 1 can corn, drained

- 1 bell pepper (any colour), diced
- 1/2 cup salsa
- 1 tablespoon chilli powder
- 1 teaspoon cumin
- 1/2 teaspoon smoked paprika
- 1/4 cup chopped fresh cilantro
- Avocado slices and lime wedges (optional)

Instructions:

- Heat olive oil in a large skillet over medium heat. Brown the ground turkey, breaking it up with a spoon.
- Add onion and garlic, and cook until softened.
- Stir in black beans, corn, bell pepper, salsa, chilli powder, cumin, smoked paprika, salt, and pepper. Simmer for 10 minutes.
- Garnish with chopped cilantro, avocado slices, and lime wedges before serving.

Ingredients:

- 1 lb ground turkey
- 1 onion, diced
- 2 cloves garlic, minced
- 14.5 oz can diced tomatoes, undrained
- 1/2 cup chopped fresh basil
- 1/4 cup chopped fresh parsley
- 1 teaspoon dried oregano

- 1/2 cup shredded mozzarella cheese
- 1/4 cup grated Parmesan cheese
- Olive oil
- Salt and pepper

Instructions:

- Preheat oven to 400°F (200°C).
- Heat olive oil in a large skillet over medium heat. Brown the ground turkey, breaking it up with a spoon.
- Add onion and garlic, and cook until softened.
- Stir in diced tomatoes, basil, parsley, oregano, salt, and pepper. Simmer for 10 minutes.
- Transfer the mixture to a baking dish. Top with mozzarella and Parmesan cheese.
- Bake for 10-15 minutes or until the cheese is melted and bubbly.

Tips:

Serve the turkey and vegetable skillet over rice, pasta, or quinoa.

Get creative with the vegetables! Add in spinach, mushrooms, or any other veggies you like.

Adjust the amount of spices to your desired level of heat.

Leftovers can be stored in an airtight container in the refrigerator for up to 3 days.

Lemon Herb Grilled Shrimp

Lemon herb grilled shrimp sounds like a fantastic dinner option! It's simple, flavorful, and perfect for a quick weeknight meal or a summer barbecue.

Classic Lemon Herb:
Ingredients:

- 1 lb large shrimp, peeled and deveined
- 2 tablespoons olive oil
- 2 tablespoons lemon juice
- 1 tablespoon chopped fresh parsley
- 1 tablespoon chopped fresh dill
- 1/2 teaspoon dried thyme
- 1/4 teaspoon salt
- 1/4 teaspoon black pepper

Instructions:

- Whisk together olive oil, lemon juice, parsley, dill, thyme, salt, and pepper in a bowl.
- Add the shrimp to the bowl and toss to coat.
- Marinate for at least 30 minutes or overnight for deeper flavour.
- Preheat the grill to medium-high heat.
- Thread the shrimp onto skewers (optional).

- Grill the shrimp for 2-3 minutes per side or until cooked through and opaque.
- Serve immediately with lemon wedges if desired.

Mediterranean Twist:

Add chopped Kalamata olives and crumbled feta cheese to the marinade for a salty and tangy touch.

Serve with grilled pita bread and hummus for a complete meal.

Spicy Kick:

Add a pinch of red pepper flakes or chopped chilli peppers to the marinade for a touch of heat.

Serve with a dollop of spicy yoghurt dip for added flavour.

Tropical Vibes:

Add chopped pineapple chunks to the marinade for a sweet and fruity twist.

Serve with grilled mango salsa for a vibrant and refreshing combination.

Additional Tips:

Use wooden skewers for a classic look, but metal skewers are easier to turn and clean.

Soak the skewers in water for at least 30 minutes to prevent burning on the grill.

Don't overcrowd the grill for even cooking.

Adjust the cooking time depending on the size of your shrimp.

Get creative with your herb and spice combinations! There are endless possibilities to explore.

Baked Sweet Potato Fries

Baked sweet potato fries! A crispy, healthy, and satisfying snack or side dish that everyone loves.

Classic and Crispy:

Ingredients:

- 2 large sweet potatoes, peeled and cut into thick wedges
- 1 tablespoon olive oil
- 1/2 teaspoon salt
- 1/4 teaspoon black pepper

Instructions:

- Preheat oven to 425°F (220°C). Line a baking sheet with parchment paper.
- Toss sweet potato wedges with olive oil, salt, and pepper.
- Spread the wedges in a single layer on the prepared baking sheet.
- Bake for 20-25 minutes, flipping halfway through, until golden brown and tender-crisp.

- Serve immediately with your favourite dipping sauce.

Spicy Kick:

Add a pinch of cayenne pepper or paprika to the seasoning mix for a touch of heat.

Drizzle with sriracha or sriracha mayo for an extra spicy kick.

Garlic Parmesan:

Toss the sweet potato wedges with a mixture of olive oil, garlic powder, Parmesan cheese, and dried oregano before baking.

Sprinkle with additional Parmesan cheese after baking for even more flavour.

Sweet and Savory:

Drizzle the baked fries with a mixture of honey and Dijon mustard for a sweet and savoury twist.

Sprinkle with chopped pecans or walnuts for added crunch and texture.

Mediterranean Vibes:

Toss the sweet potato wedges with a mixture of olive oil, lemon juice, dried oregano, rosemary, and thyme before baking.

Serve with crumbled feta cheese, olives, and chopped fresh parsley.

Tips:

Use thick wedges for the best crispy texture.

Don't overcrowd the baking sheet! This will prevent even browning and crisping.

Use sweet potatoes with bright orange flesh for the sweetest flavour.

Get creative with your dipping sauces! Try guacamole, hummus, ranch dressing, or even a simple yoghurt dip with herbs.

No matter how you choose to prepare them, baked sweet potato fries are a delicious and healthy way to enjoy this versatile vegetable. So grab your sweet potatoes and get creative! I hope these variations inspire you to whip up a batch of crispy and satisfying fries.

Salmon and Avocado Salad

Salmon and avocado salad – a match made in heaven! It's perfect for a light and refreshing lunch, a satisfying dinner, or even as a starter for a special occasion.

Mediterranean Inspired:

Ingredients:

- 4 oz cooked salmon, flaked
- 1 avocado, diced

- 1 cup cherry tomatoes, halved
- 1/2 cucumber, diced
- 1/4 cup red onion, thinly sliced
- 1/4 cup crumbled feta cheese
- 2 tablespoons olive oil
- 1 tablespoon lemon juice
- 1/2 teaspoon dried oregano
- 1/4 teaspoon salt
- 1/4 teaspoon black pepper
- Chopped fresh parsley for garnish (optional)

Instructions:

Combine all ingredients in a large bowl, except for the parsley.

Toss gently to coat.

Garnish with fresh parsley (optional) and serve immediately.

Asian Twist:

Ingredients:

- 4 oz cooked salmon, flaked
- 1 avocado, diced
- 1 cup shredded cabbage
- 1/2 cup carrot, shredded
- 1/4 cup sliced radishes
- 2 tablespoons sesame oil

- 1 tablespoon soy sauce
- 1 tablespoon rice vinegar
- 1 teaspoon honey
- 1/2 teaspoon ginger powder
- 1/4 teaspoon sriracha (optional)
- Sesame seeds, for garnish (optional)

Instructions:

- Combine all ingredients in a large bowl, except for the sesame seeds.
- Toss gently to coat.
- Garnish with sesame seeds (optional) and serve immediately.

Tips:

Use leftover cooked salmon, or you can bake, grill, or pan-sear fresh salmon as desired.

Adjust the amount of vegetables and herbs to your liking.

Get creative with your dressing! You can use other bases like Greek yoghurt, tahini, or even vinaigrette.

Serve the salad on a bed of lettuce or rice for a more substantial meal.

This salad is also great for meal prep – simply store it in an airtight container in the refrigerator for up to 3 days.

Spaghetti Squash with Tomato Sauce

spaghetti squash with tomato sauce – a classic veggie-based comfort food that's both delicious and healthy!

Simple and Easy:

Ingredients:

- 1 large spaghetti squash (around 4-5 pounds)
- 1 tablespoon olive oil
- 1 onion, chopped
- 2 cloves garlic, minced
- 1 (14.5 oz) can of diced tomatoes, undrained
- 1/2 teaspoon dried oregano
- 1/4 teaspoon salt
- 1/4 teaspoon black pepper
- Fresh basil leaves, for garnish (optional)

Instructions:

- Preheat oven to 400°F (200°C). Line a baking sheet with parchment paper.
- Cut the spaghetti squash in half lengthwise and scoop out the seeds. Brush the insides with olive oil.
- Place the squash halves, cut-side down, on the prepared baking sheet. Bake for 30-40 minutes or until tender when pierced with a fork.

- Meanwhile, heat olive oil in a large skillet over medium heat. Add onion and cook until softened about 5 minutes.
- Add garlic and cook for another minute until fragrant.
- Stir in diced tomatoes, oregano, salt, and pepper. Bring to a simmer and cook for 10 minutes.
- When the squash is cooked, use a fork to scrape the flesh into strands.
- Add the spaghetti squash strands to the tomato sauce and toss to combine.
- Garnish with fresh basil leaves (optional) and serve immediately.

Mediterranean Vibes:

Add chopped sun-dried tomatoes, Kalamata olives, and crumbled feta cheese to the finished dish for a salty and tangy twist.

Substitute fresh herbs like basil, oregano, and thyme with dried herbs for a bolder flavour.

Spicy Kick:

Add a pinch of red pepper flakes or chopped chilli peppers to the tomato sauce for a touch of heat.

Serve with a dollop of hot sauce or spicy yoghurt dip for an extra fiery kick.

Hearty Additions:

Stir in cooked ground turkey, sausage, or lentils to the tomato sauce for added protein and substance.

Add in chopped spinach or kale for extra vitamins and greens.

Creamy Delight:

Stir in a couple of tablespoons of ricotta cheese or Greek yoghurt to the tomato sauce for a richer and creamier texture.

Drizzle with pesto or a sprinkle of Parmesan cheese for a more decadent dish.

Tips:

Use a sharp knife to easily cut through the spaghetti squash.

Don't overcrowd the baking sheet when roasting the squash.

Adjust the cooking time depending on the size of your squash.

Get creative with your toppings! Chopped nuts, seeds, avocado slices, or even a fried egg can add extra flavour and texture.

With its versatility and adaptability, spaghetti squash with tomato sauce is a dish you can enjoy all year round. So gather your favourite ingredients, get creative, and whip up a pot of this delicious and satisfying meal!

Chickpea and Spinach Stew

This is a hearty and flavorful stew that is perfect for a cold day. It is packed with protein and fibre from the chickpeas and vitamins and minerals from the spinach. It is also very easy to make and can be made in under an hour.

Ingredients:

- 1 tablespoon olive oil
- 1 onion, chopped
- 2 cloves garlic, minced
- 1 teaspoon ground cumin
- 1/2 teaspoon smoked paprika
- 1/4 teaspoon cayenne pepper (optional)
- 1 (28-ounce) can of diced tomatoes, undrained
- 1 (15-ounce) can chickpeas, drained and rinsed
- 4 cups vegetable broth
- 10 ounces of fresh spinach
- Salt and pepper to taste

Instructions:

- Heat the olive oil in a large pot or Dutch oven over medium heat. Add the onion and cook until softened about 5 minutes. Add the garlic, cumin, paprika, and cayenne pepper (if using) and cook for 1 minute more.

- Add the diced tomatoes and their juices, chickpeas, and vegetable broth to the pot. Bring to a boil, then reduce heat to low and simmer for 20 minutes.
- Stir in the spinach and cook until wilted about 1 minute. Season with salt and pepper to taste.
- Serve hot with crusty bread or rice.

Tips:

You can use frozen spinach instead of fresh spinach. If using frozen spinach, add it to the pot in the last 5 minutes of cooking.

To make this stew vegan, use vegetable broth instead of chicken broth.

You can add other vegetables to this stew, such as carrots, celery, or potatoes.

If you like your stew spicy, you can add more cayenne pepper or a chopped jalapeno pepper.

This stew can be made ahead of time and reheated.

I hope you enjoy this delicious and easy recipe for Chickpea and Spinach Stew!

Greek Chicken Souvlaki

Greek Chicken Souvlaki! Tender, juicy chicken marinated in a symphony of Greek flavours, grilled to perfection on skewers, and then nestled in warm pita bread with a cooling dollop of tzatziki sauce. It's a quintessential street food experience, but you can easily recreate the magic at home.

Ingredients:

For the marinade:

- 1/4 cup olive oil
- 2 tablespoons lemon juice
- 2 tablespoons fresh oregano, chopped
- 1 tablespoon garlic, minced
- 1 teaspoon dried thyme
- 1/2 teaspoon salt
- 1/4 teaspoon black pepper

For the chicken:

- 1 pound boneless, skinless chicken breasts or thighs cut into 1-inch cubes

For serving:

- 4 pita breads
- Tzatziki sauce (recipe below or store-bought)
- Red onion, sliced
- Tomato, sliced
- Optional: Lettuce, crumbled feta cheese, Kalamata olives

Instructions:

- Make the marinade: Whisk together olive oil, lemon juice, oregano, garlic, thyme, salt, and pepper in a bowl.
- Marinate the chicken: Add the chicken cubes to the marinade and toss to coat. Cover and refrigerate for at least 30 minutes or up to overnight for deeper flavor.

- Prepare the skewers: Thread the marinated chicken onto the skewers.
- Grill the chicken: Preheat your grill to medium-high heat. Grill the chicken skewers for 5-7 minutes per side or until cooked through.
- Assemble the souvlaki: Warm the pita breads. Spread each pita with tzatziki sauce, then top with grilled chicken, red onion, tomato, and any other desired toppings.
- Serve and enjoy!

Tzatziki Sauce Recipe:

-
- 1 cup Greek yogurt
- 1/2 cucumber, seeded and grated
- 1 clove garlic, minced
- 1 tablespoon fresh dill, chopped

* 1 tablespoon olive oil
* 1/2 lemon, juiced
* Salt and pepper to taste

Instructions:

* Combine all ingredients in a bowl and mix well.
* Refrigerate for at least 30 minutes before serving.

Tips:

For even more flavour, marinate the chicken for longer, like overnight.

If you don't have wooden skewers, you can use metal skewers, but soak them in water for 30 minutes first to prevent burning.

Don't overcrowd the grill when cooking the chicken.

Get creative with your toppings! Kalamata olives, crumbled feta cheese, and lettuce are all popular additions.

I hope this helps you bring a taste of Greece to your table!

Eggplant Parmesan

Eggplant Parmesan is a delightful dish that combines tender, golden-brown eggplant slices with rich marinara sauce, melted mozzarella cheese, and a sprinkle of Parmesan cheese. It's a hearty and satisfying meal that's perfect for any occasion, from a casual weeknight dinner to a special weekend feast.

Here's what you'll need to whip up this Italian-American classic:

Ingredients:
For the eggplant:
- 2 large eggplants (about 1 1/2 pounds)
- 1 1/2 teaspoons salt
- 1/2 cup all-purpose flour
- 3 large eggs, beaten
- 1 1/2 cups Italian seasoned breadcrumbs
- Vegetable oil for frying (about 3 cups)
- For the sauce and assembly:
- 1 (28-ounce) can crushed tomatoes
- 1 (6-ounce) can tomato paste
- 1/2 teaspoon dried oregano
- 1/4 teaspoon dried basil
- 1/4 teaspoon garlic powder
- Pinch of red pepper flakes (optional)
- 1 (16-ounce) package of shredded mozzarella cheese
- 1/2 cup grated Parmesan cheese
- Fresh basil leaves, for garnish (optional)

Instructions:

- **Prepare the eggplant**: Slice the eggplants into 1/2-inch thick rounds. Sprinkle both sides with salt and let them sit for 30 minutes to release any bitterness. Rinse and pat dry with paper towels.
- **Set up the breading station:** Place the flour, beaten eggs, and breadcrumbs in separate shallow bowls.
- **Bread the eggplant:** Dredge each eggplant slice in the flour, then dip it in the egg, and finally coat it evenly with breadcrumbs.
- **Fry the eggplant:** Heat the oil in a large skillet or Dutch oven over medium-high heat. Fry the breaded eggplant in batches until golden brown and tender, about 3-4 minutes per side. Drain on paper towels.
- **Make the sauce:** In a saucepan, combine the crushed tomatoes, tomato paste, oregano, basil, garlic powder, and red pepper flakes (if using). Bring to a simmer and cook for 10 minutes, stirring occasionally.
- **Assemble the dish:** Preheat the oven to 400°F (200°C). Spread a thin layer of sauce on the bottom of a baking dish. Arrange the fried eggplant slices in a single layer and top with sauce, mozzarella cheese, and a sprinkle of Parmesan cheese. Repeat with another layer of eggplant, sauce, cheese, and Parmesan.

- **Bake and serve:** Bake for 20-25 minutes or until the cheese is melted and bubbly. Garnish with fresh basil leaves, if desired, and serve hot with crusty bread or pasta.

Tips:

You can bake the eggplant instead of frying it for a healthier option. Preheat the oven to 400°F (200°C) and brush the eggplant slices with olive oil. Bake for 20-25 minutes or until tender and golden brown.

To make the dish ahead of time, assemble it and bake it as directed. Then, let it cool completely and store it in the refrigerator for up to 2 days. Reheat in the oven before serving.

Feel free to get creative with the toppings! You can add other vegetables like zucchini or mushrooms or a drizzle of balsamic glaze for added sweetness.

Eggplant Parmesan is a versatile dish that can be easily adapted to your preferences. So, get cooking and enjoy this delicious and comforting classic!

Black Bean and Corn Salad

Black bean and corn salad is a simple, healthy, and refreshing dish that is perfect for a summer day. It is made with black beans, corn, tomatoes, red onion, cilantro, and a lime vinaigrette. It is a great side dish for grilled chicken or fish, or it can be served as a main course.

Here are the ingredients for black bean and corn salad:

- 1 (15-ounce) can black beans, drained and rinsed
- 1 (15-ounce) can corn, drained
- 1 cup chopped tomatoes
- 1/2 cup chopped red onion
- 1/4 cup chopped cilantro

For the lime vinaigrette:
- 2 tablespoons olive oil
- 2 tablespoons lime juice
- 1 teaspoon honey
- 1/2 teaspoon salt
- 1/4 teaspoon black pepper

Instructions:
- In a large bowl, combine the black beans, corn, tomatoes, red onion, and cilantro.
- In a small bowl, whisk together the olive oil, lime juice, honey, salt, and pepper.
- Pour the vinaigrette over the salad and toss to coat.
- Serve immediately.

Tips:

You can use fresh or frozen corn in this recipe.

If you don't have fresh cilantro, you can use 1 tablespoon of dried cilantro.

To make this salad more filling, you can add cooked chicken or shrimp.

This salad can be stored in the refrigerator for up to 3 days.

Here are some variations of black bean and corn salad:

Avocado Black Bean and Corn Salad: Add 1 diced avocado to the salad.

Spicy Black Bean and Corn Salad: Add 1/2 teaspoon of chilli powder or 1 chopped jalapeno pepper to the salad.

Black Bean and Corn Salad with Fajita Veggies: Add 1/2 cup of chopped bell peppers and 1/4 cup of chopped red onion to the salad.

I hope you enjoy this recipe for black bean and corn salad! It is a great way to get your daily dose of vegetables and protein.

Cauliflower and Broccoli Gratin

Cauliflower and broccoli gratin is a delightful dish that showcases the beauty of simple, fresh ingredients. The tender florets bathed in a rich, cheesy sauce and topped with a golden breadcrumbs crust are a guaranteed crowd-pleaser. It's perfect for a comforting side dish or a light vegetarian main course.

Ingredients:

- 1 head cauliflower, cut into florets
- 1 head broccoli, cut into florets
- 4 tablespoons unsalted butter
- 4 tablespoons all-purpose flour
- 4 cups milk
- 2 cups grated Gruyère cheese
- 1/2 cup grated Parmesan cheese
- 1/4 teaspoon freshly grated nutmeg
- Salt and freshly ground black pepper to taste
- 1/2 cup panko breadcrumbs
- 2 tablespoons grated Parmesan cheese
- 2 tablespoons chopped fresh parsley (optional)

Instructions:

- Preheat oven to 400°F (200°C). Lightly grease a 9x13-inch baking dish.
- Bring a large pot of salted water to a boil. Add the cauliflower and broccoli florets and blanch for 3-4 minutes or until slightly tender-crisp. Drain well and set aside.

- In a medium saucepan, melt butter over medium heat. Whisk in flour and cook for 1 minute, stirring constantly.
- Gradually whisk in milk and bring to a simmer. Cook, stirring constantly, until sauce thickens, about 5 minutes.
- Remove from heat and stir in Gruyère cheese, Parmesan cheese, nutmeg, salt, and pepper.
- In a small bowl, combine panko breadcrumbs with Parmesan cheese and parsley (if using).
- Arrange the blanched cauliflower and broccoli florets in a single layer in the prepared baking dish. Pour the cheese sauce over the vegetables, making sure to coat them evenly.
- Sprinkle the breadcrumb mixture over the top.
- Bake for 20-25 minutes or until golden brown and bubbly.
- Let cool slightly before serving.

Tips:

For a richer flavour, use heavy cream instead of milk.

You can add other vegetables to the gratin, such as sliced onions, zucchini, or mushrooms.

If you don't have Gruyère cheese, you can substitute it with sharp cheddar cheese.

Leftovers can be stored in an airtight container in the refrigerator for up to 3 days. Reheat in the oven until warmed through.

Enjoy this simple yet satisfying cauliflower and broccoli gratin! It's a healthy and delicious way to get your daily dose of vegetables.

Lentil and Vegetable Stir-Fry

Lentil and vegetable stir-fry is a fantastic, hearty, and flavorful dish that's perfect for a quick and easy weeknight meal. It's packed with protein and fiber from the lentils, vitamins and minerals from the vegetables, and can be easily customized to your preferences.

Here's what you'll need to whip up this healthy and delicious stir-fry:

Ingredients:

- 1 cup dried lentils, rinsed
- 2 tablespoons olive oil
- 1 onion, chopped
- 2 cloves garlic, minced
- 1 red bell pepper, sliced
- 1 green bell pepper, sliced
- 1 carrot, sliced
- 1 zucchini, sliced

- 1/2 cup vegetable broth
- 1/4 cup soy sauce
- 1 tablespoon rice vinegar
- 1 teaspoon Sriracha (optional)
- 1/2 teaspoon ground ginger
- Salt and pepper to taste
- Cooked brown rice, quinoa, or couscous for serving
- Chopped fresh cilantro for garnish (optional)

Instructions:

Cook the lentils according to package instructions. Drain and set aside.

Heat olive oil in a large wok or skillet over medium-high heat. Add the onion and cook until softened about 5 minutes.

Add the garlic, bell peppers, and carrot, and cook for another 3-4 minutes or until the vegetables are slightly tender-crisp.

Stir in the zucchini and cook for another minute.

Add the vegetable broth, soy sauce, rice vinegar, Sriracha (if using), and ginger. Bring to a simmer and cook for 2-3 minutes or until the sauce is slightly thickened.

Stir in the cooked lentils and heat through. Season with salt and pepper to taste.

Serve the lentil and vegetable stir-fry over cooked brown rice, quinoa, or couscous. Garnish with chopped fresh cilantro, if desired.

Tips:

Feel free to get creative with the vegetables! You can add other favourites like broccoli, mushrooms, or snow peas.

If you don't have vegetable broth, you can use water.

For a thicker sauce, you can add a cornstarch slurry (1 tablespoon cornstarch mixed with 2 tablespoons water) to the pan before adding the lentils.

Leftovers can be stored in an airtight container in the refrigerator for up to 3 days. Reheat gently in a pan or microwave.

Here are some additional variations you can try:

Spicy Lentil and Vegetable Stir-Fry: Add 1/2 teaspoon of red pepper flakes to the pan with the garlic.

Thai Lentil and Vegetable Stir-Fry: Add 1 tablespoon of Thai curry paste to the pan with the garlic.

Indian Lentil and Vegetable Stir-Fry: Add 1 teaspoon of garam masala to the pan with the garlic.

I hope you enjoy this recipe for lentil and vegetable stir-fry! It's a healthy, flavorful, and satisfying meal that's perfect for any occasion.

<h1 style="text-align:center">Shrimp and Quinoa Bowl</h1>

Shrimp and quinoa bowls are a fantastic way to enjoy a healthy, delicious, and customizable meal. With the base of protein-rich quinoa and succulent shrimp, you can layer on flavours with various vegetables, sauces, and toppings to create your own personal masterpiece. Here's a basic guide to get you started:

Ingredients:

For the quinoa:

- 1 cup quinoa, rinsed
- 1 1/2 cups water or vegetable broth

For the shrimp:

- 1 pound shrimp, peeled and deveined
- 1 tablespoon olive oil
- 1/2 teaspoon salt
- 1/4 teaspoon black pepper
- 1/4 teaspoon paprika (optional)

For the vegetables (choose 2-3):

- Chopped avocado
- Diced tomatoes
- Sliced cucumber
- Shredded carrots
- Steamed broccoli or asparagus

- Roasted sweet potato cubes

For the sauces (choose 1-2):

- Cilantro lime crema (mix Greek yoghurt with lime juice, chopped cilantro, salt, and pepper)
- Sesame ginger dressing (whisk together soy sauce, rice vinegar, sesame oil, grated ginger, honey, and sriracha)
- Avocado crema (blend avocado with a squeeze of lemon juice, salt, and pepper)

For the toppings (choose 2-3):

- Chopped fresh herbs (cilantro, parsley, mint)
- Crumbled feta cheese
- Pumpkin seeds
- Sliced almonds
- Hot sauce

Instructions:

- **Cook the quinoa:** Rinse the quinoa and add it to a saucepan with water or broth. Bring to a boil, then reduce heat, cover, and simmer for 15 minutes or until fluffy. Fluff with a fork and set aside.
- **Marinate the shrimp:** In a bowl, combine shrimp with olive oil, salt, pepper, and paprika (optional). Marinate for 10 minutes if desired.

- **Cook the shrimp:** Heat a large skillet or grill pan over medium-high heat. Add the shrimp and cook until pink and opaque, about 2-3 minutes per side.
- **Assemble the bowls:** Divide the cooked quinoa into individual bowls. Top with your chosen vegetables, shrimp, sauce(s), and toppings.
- Enjoy! Customize your bowl to your taste and savour the flavours.

Tips:

Feel free to get creative with the ingredients! Use any vegetables, sauces, and toppings you like.

Leftovers can be stored in airtight containers in the refrigerator for up to 3 days. Reheat the quinoa and shrimp gently before serving.

This recipe is easily adapted for different dietary needs. For a vegetarian option, omit the shrimp and add tofu or black beans. For a vegan option, use vegetable broth for the quinoa and a vegan-friendly sauce.

Here are some additional flavour variations you can try:

Mediterranean Bowl: Add roasted red peppers, Kalamata olives, feta cheese, and a Greek yoghurt sauce.

Spicy Thai Bowl: Use a sweet chilli sauce for the dressing, add chopped mango, and top with crushed peanuts.

Tropical Bowl: Add pineapple chunks, shredded coconut, and a mango salsa.

I hope this inspires you to create your own delicious shrimp and quinoa bowl! Don't hesitate to experiment and find your perfect combination of flavours.

Stuffed Acorn Squash with Quinoa and Cranberries

Acorn squash, filled with a warm autumnal blend of quinoa, cranberries, and savoury spices, is a delightful dish perfect for a cosy fall meal. It's a vegetarian feast for the senses, offering vibrant colours, contrasting textures, and a symphony of sweet and savoury flavours.

Ingredients:

For the squash:

- 2 medium acorn squash
- 1 tablespoon olive oil
- 1/2 teaspoon salt
- 1/4 teaspoon black pepper

For the filling:

- 1 cup cooked quinoa
- 1/2 cup dried cranberries
- 1/2 cup chopped onion

- 1/2 cup chopped apple (such as Granny Smith)
- 2 cloves garlic, minced
- 1/2 cup chopped walnuts
- 1/2 teaspoon dried sage
- 1/4 teaspoon dried thyme
- 1/4 teaspoon salt
- 1/4 teaspoon black pepper
- 1/4 cup vegetable broth
- 1/4 cup maple syrup (optional)

Instructions:

- Preheat oven to 400°F (200°C).
- **Prepare the squash:** Cut the acorn squash in half lengthwise and scoop out the seeds and membranes. Drizzle each half with olive oil, season with salt and pepper, and place cut-side down on a baking sheet. Roast for 20-25 minutes or until tender-crisp.
- **Cook the quinoa:** While the squash roasts, cook the quinoa according to package instructions. Set aside to cool slightly.
- **Make the filling:** Heat a tablespoon of olive oil in a skillet over medium heat. Add the onion and cook until softened about 5 minutes. Add the apple and garlic, and cook for another 2 minutes.
- Stir in the cooked quinoa, cranberries, walnuts, sage, thyme, salt, pepper, and vegetable broth. Cook for 2-

3 minutes, until heated through. If desired, add a drizzle of maple syrup for a touch of sweetness.

- **Assemble and bake:** Fill the roasted squash halves with the quinoa mixture. Bake for an additional 10-15 minutes or until heated through and golden brown on top.
- Serve and enjoy! Garnish with fresh herbs like parsley or sage and a sprinkle of additional chopped walnuts if desired.

Tips:

For extra flavour, toast the walnuts in a dry pan before adding them to the filling.

You can substitute pecans or almonds for the walnuts.

If you don't have apples, you can use other fruits like chopped pear or dried apricots.

Leftovers can be stored in an airtight container in the refrigerator for up to 3 days. Reheat gently in the oven or microwave.

This recipe is a versatile canvas for your culinary creativity. Feel free to add other vegetables like chopped mushrooms or shredded carrots, or try different herbs like rosemary or oregano. Get creative and enjoy the delightful combination of textures and flavours in this autumnal masterpiece!

Cabbage and Apple Slaw

Cabbage and apple slaw is a refreshing and versatile salad that can be enjoyed as a side dish, topping, or even a light meal. The crunchy cabbage pairs beautifully with the sweet and tart apples, while a flavorful dressing brings it all together. Here are a few recipe variations to get you started:

Basic Cabbage and Apple Slaw:
Ingredients:

- 1/2 head of green cabbage, thinly sliced
- 1 apple (Granny Smith or Honeycrisp recommended), thinly sliced
- 1/4 cup mayonnaise
- 2 tablespoons apple cider vinegar
- 1 teaspoon Dijon mustard
- 1/2 teaspoon honey
- Salt and pepper to taste

Instructions:

- Combine the cabbage and apple in a large bowl.
- Whisk together the mayonnaise, apple cider vinegar, Dijon mustard, and honey in a small bowl.
- Pour the dressing over the cabbage and apple mixture and toss to coat.
- Season with salt and pepper to taste.

- Serve immediately, or refrigerate for at least 30 minutes for the flavours to meld.

Variations:

- **Creamy Slaw:** Add 1/4 cup of sour cream or plain Greek yoghurt to the dressing for a richer creaminess.
- **Spicy Slaw**: Add a pinch of red pepper flakes or chilli powder to the dressing for a kick.
- **Tropical Slaw:** Add chopped pineapple, mango, and toasted coconut flakes for a tropical twist.
- **Asian Slaw:** Use rice vinegar instead of apple cider vinegar, and add a teaspoon of grated ginger and a drizzle of sesame oil to the dressing.
- **Waldorf Slaw**: Add chopped celery, grapes, and walnuts for a classic Waldorf salad twist.

Tips:

Use a mandoline or food processor for quick and even slicing of the cabbage and apple.

If you don't have Dijon mustard, you can substitute regular mustard.

For a vegan slaw, use vegan mayonnaise and yoghurt alternatives.

Leftovers can be stored in an airtight container in the refrigerator for up to 3 days, but the apples may brown slightly.

No matter your preference, there's a delicious cabbage and apple slaw variation out there for you. Get creative, experiment with different ingredients and flavours, and enjoy this refreshing and healthy salad!

Grilled Turkey Burgers

Grilled turkey burgers are a fantastic alternative to their beefy counterparts, offering a leaner and flavour-packed option for your summer BBQs or weeknight dinners. Packed with moisture and seasoned just right, they can be just as satisfying and delicious as a classic burger. Here's how to create your own juicy turkey burger masterpiece:

Ingredients:

For the patties:

- 1 pound ground turkey (ideally 85/15 lean-to-fat ratio)
- 1/2 cup breadcrumbs
- 1/4 cup finely chopped onion
- 1/4 cup finely chopped bell pepper (your choice of colour)
- 2 cloves garlic, minced
- 1 egg, beaten

- 1 tablespoon olive oil
- 1/2 teaspoon dried oregano
- 1/2 teaspoon dried thyme
- 1/4 teaspoon salt
- 1/4 teaspoon black pepper

For the toppings (choose your favourites):
- Hamburger buns
- Lettuce
- Tomato
- Onion
- Pickle
- Cheese (cheddar, swiss, pepper jack, etc.)
- Mustard
- Ketchup
- Mayonnaise
- Aioli
- BBQ sauce
- Guacamole
- Any other creative toppings you can imagine!

Instructions:

- Combine the turkey burger ingredients: In a large bowl, mix together the ground turkey, breadcrumbs, onion, bell pepper, garlic, egg, olive oil, oregano, thyme, salt, and pepper. Gently mix until just combined, taking care not to overwork the meat.

- Form the patties: Divide the mixture into 4 equal portions and shape them into patties slightly larger than your hamburger buns. Make a thumbprint indentation in the centre of each patty to prevent them from bulging in the middle while cooking.
- Preheat your grill: Heat your grill to medium-high heat (around 400°F). If using a charcoal grill, wait until the coals are hot and white.
- Grill the burgers: Place the turkey burgers on the preheated grill and cook for 4-5 minutes per side or until cooked through to an internal temperature of 165°F.
- Assemble and enjoy! Toast your hamburger buns while the burgers cook. Then, build your burger masterpieces with your chosen toppings and savour the juicy, flavorful goodness!

Tips:

For extra moisture and flavour, mix in a grated zucchini or finely chopped apple to the turkey burger mixture.

Don't press down on the patties while grilling! This can squeeze out the juices and make them dry.

Get creative with your toppings! The possibilities are endless, so experiment and find your perfect combination.

Leftover turkey burgers can be stored in an airtight container in the refrigerator for up to 3 days. Reheat gently in a pan or microwave.

Grilled turkey burgers are a versatile and delicious way to enjoy a healthy and satisfying meal. With the right ingredients and some simple tips, you can create juicy, flavorful burgers that will rival any beef burger out there. So get grilling and enjoy!

CHAPTER 8
Mango Salsa Chicken

Mango salsa chicken is a vibrant and flavorful dish that's perfect for a light and refreshing summer meal. The sweet and tangy mango salsa pairs beautifully with the tender chicken, creating a symphony of contrasting flavours and textures. Here are two delicious options for you to try:

Option 1: Baked Mango Salsa Chicken:
Ingredients:

- 4 boneless, skinless chicken breasts
- 1/2 cup fresh mango, diced
- 1/4 cup red onion, finely diced
- 1/4 cup cilantro, chopped
- 1 tablespoon lime juice
- 1 teaspoon olive oil
- 1/2 teaspoon salt
- 1/4 teaspoon black pepper
- 1/4 cup shredded mozzarella cheese (optional)

Instructions:
- Preheat oven to 400°F (200°C).

- Combine the mango, red onion, cilantro, lime juice, olive oil, salt, and pepper in a bowl.
- Place the chicken breasts in a baking dish. Spread the mango salsa evenly over the chicken.
- Bake for 20-25 minutes, or until the chicken is cooked through and the salsa is bubbly.
- Top with shredded mozzarella cheese (optional) and broil for 1-2 minutes, until golden brown and melted.
- Serve with your favourite sides, such as rice, quinoa, or roasted vegetables.

Option 2: Grilled Mango Salsa Chicken:

Ingredients:
- 4 boneless, skinless chicken breasts
- 1/2 cup fresh mango, diced
- 1/4 cup red onion, finely diced
- 1/4 cup cilantro, chopped
- 1 tablespoon lime juice
- 1 teaspoon olive oil
- 1/2 teaspoon salt
- 1/4 teaspoon black pepper
- 4 skewers

Instructions:

- Combine the mango, red onion, cilantro, lime juice, olive oil, salt, and pepper in a bowl.
- Thread the chicken breasts onto skewers.
- Preheat your grill to medium-high heat.
- Brush the chicken with the mango salsa mixture.
- Grill the chicken for 5-7 minutes per side or until cooked through and the salsa is slightly caramelized.
- Serve with your favourite sides, such as grilled vegetables, corn tortillas, or avocado slices.

Tips:

You can use frozen mango chunks in a pinch, but fresh mango will have a brighter flavour.

If you don't have cilantro, you can substitute parsley or mint.

For a spicier version, add a pinch of chilli flakes or chopped jalapeno to the salsa.

Leftovers can be stored in an airtight container in the refrigerator for up to 3 days. Reheat gently in a pan or microwave.

No matter which option you choose, you're sure to enjoy the fresh and flavorful goodness of mango salsa chicken. So get cooking and savour the taste of summer!

Vegetable and Lentil Soup

Vegetable and lentil soup is a hearty, healthy, and flavorful dish that's perfect for a cosy autumn or winter meal. It's packed with protein and fiber from the lentils, vitamins and minerals from the vegetables, and can be easily customized to your taste with different vegetables, spices, and herbs. Here's a basic blueprint to get you started:

Ingredients:

- 1 tablespoon olive oil
- 1 onion, chopped
- 2 carrots, chopped
- 2 celery stalks, chopped
- 2 cloves garlic, minced
- 1 cup dried lentils, rinsed
- 4 cups vegetable broth
- Four cups chopped vegetables (choose 3-4): Bell peppers, broccoli, mushrooms, kale, spinach, potatoes, etc.
- 1 (14.5 oz) can of diced tomatoes, undrained
- 1 teaspoon dried thyme
- 1/2 teaspoon dried oregano
- Salt and pepper to taste
- Optional garnishes: Chopped fresh parsley, grated parmesan cheese, crusty bread

Instructions:

- Heat olive oil in a large pot or Dutch oven over medium heat. Add onion, carrots, and celery, and cook until softened, about 5 minutes.
- Add garlic and cook for another minute until fragrant.
- Stir in lentils, vegetable broth, tomatoes, thyme, and oregano. Bring to a boil, then reduce heat, cover, and simmer for 20 minutes or until lentils are tender.
- Add your chosen chopped vegetables and continue simmering for another 10-15 minutes or until vegetables are tender-crisp.
- Season with salt and pepper to taste.
- Serve hot, garnished with chopped fresh parsley, grated parmesan cheese, and crusty bread (optional).

Tips:

Feel free to get creative with the vegetables! You can use any vegetables you like or even add cooked grains like quinoa or brown rice.

For a thicker soup, mash some of the cooked lentils against the side of the pot with a fork.

If you don't have vegetable broth, you can use water and add 1 tablespoon of vegetable bouillon powder.

Leftovers can be stored in an airtight container in the refrigerator for up to 3 days. Reheat gently in a pot or microwave.

Here are some additional variations you can try:

Spicy Vegetable and Lentil Soup: Add a pinch of red pepper flakes or chilli powder to the pot with the garlic.

Curried Vegetable and Lentil Soup: Add 1 tablespoon of curry powder to the pot with the garlic.

Coconut Curry Vegetable and Lentil Soup: Use coconut milk instead of vegetable broth for a creamy and flavorful twist.

I hope this recipe inspires you to create your own delicious vegetable and lentil soup! It's a versatile and comforting dish that everyone will enjoy.

Roasted Brussels Sprouts with Balsamic Glaze

Roasted Brussels sprouts with balsamic glaze is a classic and delicious side dish that's perfect for elevating any meal. The caramelized Brussels sprouts with a touch of sweet and tangy balsamic glaze are a surefire crowd-pleaser. Here are two versions you can try:

Option 1: Simple Roasted Brussels Sprouts with Balsamic Glaze:

Ingredients:

- 1 1/2 pounds Brussels sprouts, trimmed and halved
- 2 tablespoons olive oil
- 1/2 teaspoon salt
- 1/4 teaspoon black pepper
- 1/4 cup balsamic vinegar
- 1 tablespoon honey (optional)

Instructions:

- Preheat oven to 400°F (200°C).
- Toss the Brussels sprouts with olive oil, salt, and pepper in a large bowl.
- Spread the Brussels sprouts in an even layer on a baking sheet.
- Roast for 20-25 minutes or until tender and lightly browned.
- While the Brussels sprouts are roasting, heat the balsamic vinegar in a small saucepan over medium heat. Bring to a simmer and cook until reduced by half and slightly thickened, about 5-7 minutes.
- If desired, stir in the honey and cook for another minute to blend.
- Drizzle the balsamic glaze over the roasted Brussels sprouts and serve immediately.

Option 2: Maple Sriracha Roasted Brussels Sprouts with Balsamic Reduction:

Ingredients:

- 1 1/2 pounds Brussels sprouts, trimmed and halved
- 2 tablespoons olive oil
- 1/2 teaspoon salt
- 1/4 teaspoon black pepper
- 1/4 cup balsamic vinegar
- 1 tablespoon maple syrup
- 1/2 teaspoon sriracha
- 1/4 cup chopped walnuts (optional)

Instructions:

- Preheat oven to 400°F (200°C).
- Toss the Brussels sprouts with olive oil, salt, and pepper in a large bowl.
- Spread the Brussels sprouts in an even layer on a baking sheet.
- Roast for 20-25 minutes or until tender and lightly browned.
- While the Brussels sprouts are roasting, heat the balsamic vinegar in a small saucepan over medium heat. Bring to a simmer and cook until reduced by half and slightly thickened, about 5-7 minutes.
- Stir in the maple syrup and sriracha and cook for another minute to blend.

- Drizzle the balsamic reduction over the roasted Brussels sprouts and top with chopped walnuts (optional).
- Serve immediately.

Tips:

For extra crispy Brussels sprouts, cut them into smaller pieces.

You can use a variety of other sweeteners besides honey or maple syrup, such as brown sugar or agave nectar.

If you don't like spicy food, you can omit the sriracha or use a smaller amount.

Leftovers can be stored in an airtight container in the refrigerator for up to 3 days. Reheat gently in a pan or microwave.

No matter which option you choose, roasted Brussels sprouts with balsamic glaze are a simple yet delicious way to add a touch of elegance to any meal. Get creative and experiment with different flavours and toppings to find your perfect combination!

Tuna and White Bean Salad

Tuna and White Bean Salad: A Delicious and Easy Summer Recipe

Tuna and white bean salad is a light, refreshing, and protein-packed dish that's perfect for a quick lunch, picnics, or as a side dish. The combination of flaky tuna, creamy white beans, crunchy vegetables, and a flavorful dressing creates a symphony of textures and flavours that's sure to please. Here are two variations to get you started:

Option 1: Mediterranean Tuna and White Bean Salad:

Ingredients:

- 1 (15-ounce) can cannellini beans, rinsed and drained
- 1 (5-ounce) can chunk light tuna in olive oil, drained
- 1/2 cucumber, chopped
- 1/2 red onion, finely chopped
- 1/4 cup chopped cherry tomatoes
- 1/4 cup chopped Kalamata olives
- 1/4 cup chopped fresh parsley
- 2 tablespoons olive oil
- 1 tablespoon lemon juice
- 1/2 teaspoon dried oregano
- 1/4 teaspoon salt
- 1/4 teaspoon black pepper

Instructions:

In a large bowl, combine the cannellini beans, tuna, cucumber, red onion, cherry tomatoes, Kalamata olives, and parsley.

In a small bowl, whisk together the olive oil, lemon juice, oregano, salt, and pepper.

Pour the dressing over the salad and toss to coat.

Serve immediately, or chill for at least 30 minutes for the flavours to meld.

Option 2: Asian Tuna and White Bean Salad:

Ingredients:

- 1 (15-ounce) can chickpeas, rinsed and drained
- 1 (5-ounce) can chunk light tuna in water, drained
- 1/2 red bell pepper, chopped
- 1/2 green bell pepper, chopped
- 1/4 cup chopped carrots
- 1/4 cup chopped green onions
- 1/4 cup chopped fresh cilantro
- 2 tablespoons sesame oil
- 2 tablespoons rice vinegar
- 1 tablespoon soy sauce
- 1 teaspoon grated ginger
- 1/2 teaspoon sriracha (optional)
- 1/4 teaspoon salt

- 1/4 teaspoon black pepper

Instructions:

- In a large bowl, combine the chickpeas, tuna, bell peppers, carrots, green onions, and cilantro.
- In a small bowl, whisk together the sesame oil, rice vinegar, soy sauce, ginger, sriracha (optional), salt, and pepper.
- Pour the dressing over the salad and toss to coat.
- Serve immediately, or chill for at least 30 minutes for the flavours to meld.

Tips:

You can use any type of white beans you like, such as cannellini, chickpeas, or great northern beans.

For a thicker salad, mash some of the beans with a fork before adding them to the bowl.

Feel free to add other vegetables to the salad, such as chopped celery, zucchini, or broccoli.

If you don't have fresh herbs, you can use 1 teaspoon of dried oregano for the Mediterranean option or 1 teaspoon of dried coriander for the Asian option.

Leftovers can be stored in an airtight container in the refrigerator for up to 3 days.

No matter which variation you choose, tuna and white bean salad is a quick, easy, and delicious way to enjoy a light and refreshing meal. So get creative, experiment with different flavours and textures, and find your perfect tuna and white bean salad combination!

Sesame Ginger Tofu Stir-Fry

Sesame ginger tofu stir-fry is a delightful vegetarian dish packed with vibrant flavours and textures. The crispy tofu coated in a sweet and savoury sauce, paired with crunchy vegetables, makes for a satisfying and healthy meal. Here's how to whip up this delicious stir-fry:

Ingredients:

For the tofu:

- 14 oz extra-firm tofu, drained and pressed
- 1 tablespoon cornstarch
- 1/4 teaspoon salt
- 1/4 teaspoon black pepper
- 2 tablespoons vegetable oil

For the sauce:

- 2 tablespoons soy sauce
- 1 tablespoon sesame oil
- 1 tablespoon rice vinegar
- 1 tablespoon honey or brown sugar
- 1 tablespoon grated ginger

- 1 clove garlic, minced
- 1/2 teaspoon Sriracha (optional)

For the stir-fry:

- 1 red bell pepper, sliced
- 1 green bell pepper, sliced
- 1 broccoli floret, cut into bite-sized pieces
- 1/2 cup snow peas
- 1/4 cup chopped green onions
- Cooked rice, quinoa, or noodles for serving

Instructions:

Prepare the tofu: Cut the tofu into bite-sized cubes. Toss with cornstarch, salt, and pepper.

Heat the vegetable oil in a large wok or skillet over medium-high heat. Add the tofu and cook until golden brown and crispy on all sides, about 5-7 minutes per side. Drain on paper towels.

Make the sauce: In a small bowl, whisk together the soy sauce, sesame oil, rice vinegar, honey/brown sugar, ginger, garlic, and Sriracha (if using).

Stir-fry the vegetables: Add the bell peppers, broccoli, and snow peas to the wok and stir-fry for 2-3 minutes, until slightly softened but still crisp.

Combine and serve: Add the cooked tofu and sauce to the wok and toss to coat everything evenly. Heat through for another minute.

Serve the stir-fry over cooked rice, quinoa, or noodles garnished with chopped green onions.

Tips:

For extra crispy tofu, press the tofu under a weight for at least 30 minutes before cutting.

You can use any type of vegetables you like in this stir-fry. Some other options include carrots, mushrooms, zucchini, or snap peas.

Feel free to adjust the amount of Sriracha to your spice preference.

Leftovers can be stored in an airtight container in the refrigerator for up to 3 days. Reheat gently in a pan or microwave.

This sesame ginger tofu stir-fry is a quick, easy, and versatile dish that's perfect for any night of the week. Enjoy the beautiful combination of flavours and textures, and don't be afraid to get creative with your ingredients!

Lemon Herb Quinoa Salad

Lemon herb quinoa salad is a refreshing and versatile dish perfect for a light lunch, summer picnics, or as a side to grilled dishes. The fluffy quinoa is tossed with vibrant herbs, a tangy lemon dressing, and your choice of vegetables and protein for a healthy and satisfying meal. Here's a basic recipe and some variations to spark your culinary creativity:

Ingredients:

For the quinoa:

- 1 cup quinoa, rinsed
- 1 1/2 cups water or vegetable broth

For the dressing:

- 2 tablespoons olive oil
- 1 tablespoon lemon juice
- 1/2 teaspoon Dijon mustard
- 1/4 teaspoon honey
- 1/4 teaspoon dried oregano
- 1/4 teaspoon salt
- 1/4 teaspoon black pepper

For the salad:

- 1/4 cup chopped fresh parsley
- 2 tablespoons chopped fresh mint
- 1/2 cucumber, diced
- 1/2 red onion, finely chopped
- 1/4 cup crumbled feta cheese (optional)
- 1/4 cup cherry tomatoes, halved (optional)

- Additional toppings of your choice (cooked chicken, chickpeas, avocado slices, etc.)

Instructions:

- Cook the quinoa: Combine the rinsed quinoa and water or broth in a saucepan. Bring to a boil, then reduce heat, cover, and simmer for 15 minutes, or until the quinoa is fluffy and all the liquid is absorbed. Fluff with a fork and set aside to cool slightly.
- Make the dressing: In a small bowl, whisk together the olive oil, lemon juice, Dijon mustard, honey, oregano, salt, and pepper.
- Assemble the salad: In a large bowl, combine the cooled quinoa, parsley, mint, cucumber, red onion, and feta cheese (if using). Pour the dressing over the salad and toss to coat.
- Add your preferred toppings, such as cherry tomatoes, cooked chicken, chickpeas, or avocado slices.
- Serve immediately and enjoy!

Variations:

Mediterranean Twist: Add chopped Kalamata olives, roasted red peppers, and a sprinkle of crumbled feta cheese for a Mediterranean flair.

Tropical Breeze: Toss in chopped mango, pineapple, and toasted coconut flakes for a tropical twist.

Spicy Fiesta: Add a chopped jalapeno or a pinch of red pepper flakes to the dressing for a spicy kick.

Protein Power-Up: Include cooked chicken, shrimp, or chickpeas for a more substantial meal.

Tips:

Feel free to mix and match different herbs and vegetables based on your preference and what's in season.

For a creamier dressing, add a spoonful of Greek yoghurt or tahini.

Leftovers can be stored in an airtight container in the refrigerator for up to 3 days. Reheat gently in a pan or microwave.

With its endless possibilities for customization, lemon herb quinoa salad is a dish that can be enjoyed all year round. Get creative, explore different flavours and textures, and create your own delicious and refreshing quinoa salad masterpiece!

Baked Chicken Parmesan

Baked chicken parmesan is a timeless dish that satisfies with its crispy breaded coating, juicy chicken interior, and gooey melted cheese. It's perfect for a comforting family meal, a casual get-together, or even a satisfying solo dinner. Here's how to achieve this classic in your own kitchen:

Ingredients:

For the chicken:

- 4 boneless, skinless chicken breasts (4-6 oz each)
- 1/2 cup all-purpose flour
- 1/4 teaspoon salt
- 1/4 teaspoon black pepper
- 2 large eggs, beaten
- 1 cup Italian breadcrumbs
- 1/4 cup grated Parmesan cheese
- 1/4 teaspoon dried oregano

Cooking spray

For the sauce:

- 1 (28-ounce) can crushed tomatoes
- 1/2 teaspoon dried oregano
- 1/2 teaspoon dried basil
- 1/4 teaspoon garlic powder
- 1/4 teaspoon salt
- Pinch of red pepper flakes (optional)
- 1 cup shredded mozzarella cheese

Instructions:

- Preheat oven to 400°F (200°C).

- Prepare the chicken: Pound the chicken breasts to an even thickness of about 1/2 inch. Season both sides with salt and pepper.

- Set up a breading station: Place the flour in one shallow dish, the beaten eggs in another, and the combined breadcrumbs, Parmesan cheese, and oregano in a third.

- Bread the chicken: Dip each chicken breast in the flour, then the egg, and finally the breadcrumb mixture, ensuring an even coating.

- Spray a baking sheet with cooking spray and arrange the breaded chicken in a single layer.

- Bake for 15-20 minutes or until the chicken is cooked through and golden brown.

- While the chicken is baking, prepare the sauce: In a saucepan, combine the crushed tomatoes, oregano, basil, garlic powder, salt, and red pepper flakes (if using). Bring to a simmer and cook for 5 minutes.

- Assemble the dish: Remove the chicken from the oven and spoon a generous amount of sauce over each piece. Top with shredded mozzarella cheese

- and return to the oven for 5-7 minutes or until the cheese is melted and bubbly.

- Serve immediately with your favourite sides, such as pasta, roasted vegetables, or a simple salad.

Tips:

For extra crispy chicken, fry the breaded chicken in a shallow pan of hot oil for a few minutes before baking.

You can substitute panko breadcrumbs for a lighter and flakier texture.

To make the dish ahead of time, prepare the chicken parmesan up to the point of adding the cheese. Cover and refrigerate for up to 24 hours. Bake as directed, adding the cheese and broiling for a minute if needed.

Feel free to customize the sauce with additional herbs like thyme or rosemary.

Leftovers can be stored in an airtight container in the refrigerator for up to 3 days. Reheat gently in the oven or microwave.

Baked chicken parmesan is a crowd-pleasing dish that's sure to satisfy your comfort food cravings. With its simple recipe and endless customization options, you can create your own signature version of this classic. So go ahead, grab some chicken, gather your ingredients, and get ready to bake up a delicious masterpiece!

Greek Yogurt Chicken Salad

Greek yoghurt chicken salad is a delightful twist on the traditional recipe, offering a lighter and protein-packed alternative. The tangy yoghurt replaces heavier mayonnaise, creating a vibrant and flavorful salad perfect for sandwiches, wraps, salads, or even as a dip with crackers. Here's how to whip up this healthy and delicious dish:

Ingredients:

- 2 cups cooked and shredded chicken breast (can use a rotisserie chicken)
- 1 cup plain Greek yoghurt (non-fat or 2%)
- 1/2 cup chopped celery
- 1/4 cup chopped red onion
- 1/4 cup chopped fresh dill
- 2 tablespoons lemon juice
- 1 tablespoon Dijon mustard
- 1/2 teaspoon salt
- 1/4 teaspoon black pepper

Optional additions: chopped grapes, chopped apple, toasted nuts, crumbled feta cheese

Instructions:

- Combine the cooked chicken, Greek yoghurt, celery, red onion, and dill in a large bowl.
- In a small bowl, whisk together the lemon juice, Dijon mustard, salt, and pepper.
- Pour the dressing over the chicken mixture and toss to coat.
- Taste and adjust seasonings as needed.

- Fold in any optional ingredients you'd like to add.
- Chill the salad for at least 30 minutes for the flavours to meld.
- Serve on toasted bread, wraps, salad greens, or as a dip with crackers.

Tips:

For extra flavour, marinate the cooked chicken in lemon juice, olive oil, herbs, and spices before shredding.

If you prefer a creamier salad, use more yoghurt or less chicken.

To make the salad ahead of time, store it in an airtight container in the refrigerator for up to 3 days.

Feel free to experiment with different herbs and spices like parsley, oregano, or garlic powder.

Add chopped cucumber or bell peppers for extra crunch and freshness.

Greek yoghurt chicken salad is a versatile and healthy dish that's perfect for a quick lunch, light dinner, or even a picnic. With its simple recipe and endless possibilities for customization, you can create your own version to satisfy your taste buds and dietary needs. So grab your ingredients, whip up a batch of this delicious salad, and enjoy the refreshing twist on a classic!

Vegetable and Brown Rice Casserole

Vegetable and brown rice casserole! A warm, comforting, and customizable dish perfect for any occasion. Here are a few recipe variations to inspire your culinary journey:

Classic Comfort:

Vegetables: Diced carrots, celery, and onions for that familiar base. Add peas, corn, broccoli, or mushrooms for extra texture and flavour.

Rice: Cook 1 1/2 cups brown rice with vegetable broth (around 3 cups) for a nutty and earthy note.

Sauce: Combine 1 can cream of mushroom soup with 1 cup milk, 1/2 cup shredded cheddar cheese, and a sprinkle of dried thyme for a creamy and cheesy center.

Topping: Sprinkle on additional cheddar cheese, panko breadcrumbs, or crushed crackers before baking for a golden and crunchy finish.

Mediterranean Medley:

Tips and Tricks:

- Preheat your oven to 375°F (190°C) for even baking.
- Don't be afraid to get creative with your vegetables! Any combination that sounds good to you is fair game.

- For a vegan option, replace the cheese and cream of mushroom soup with plant-based alternatives like vegan cheese and a creamy cashew sauce.
- Leftovers can be stored in an airtight container in the refrigerator for up to 3 days. Reheat gently in the oven or microwave.
- Remember, the beauty of vegetable and brown rice casserole lies in its adaptability. Explore different flavours, textures, and ingredients to create your own signature dish that warms your heart and nourishes your body. So get cooking, have fun, and enjoy!

Salmon and Quinoa Patties

Salmon and quinoa patties are a fantastic way to enjoy the nutritious benefits of both ingredients in a flavorful and versatile dish. They can be served as appetizers, main courses, or even packed for lunch. Here are a couple of delicious variations to get you started:

Mediterranean Delight:

Ingredients:

- 12 oz cooked salmon, flaked
- 1 cup cooked quinoa
- 1/2 cup chopped red onion

- 1/4 cup chopped fresh parsley
- 1/4 cup crumbled feta cheese
- 1 tablespoon lemon juice
- 1 tablespoon olive oil
- 1/2 teaspoon dried oregano
- 1/4 teaspoon salt
- 1/4 teaspoon black pepper

Instructions:

Combine all ingredients in a large bowl and mix well.

Form the mixture into 6-8 patties.

Heat a lightly oiled skillet over medium heat and cook the patties for 3-4 minutes per side or until golden brown and cooked through.

Serve with a side of tzatziki sauce, mixed greens, or roasted vegetables.

Asian Fusion:

Ingredients:

- 12 oz cooked salmon, flaked
- 1 cup cooked quinoa
- 1/2 cup chopped green bell pepper
- 1/4 cup chopped scallions
- 2 tablespoons soy sauce
- 2 tablespoons rice vinegar
- 1 tablespoon sesame oil

- 1 tablespoon grated ginger
- 1 clove garlic, minced
- 1/4 teaspoon Sriracha (optional)
- 1/4 teaspoon salt
- 1/4 teaspoon black pepper

Instructions:

- Combine all ingredients in a large bowl and mix well.
- Form the mixture into 6-8 patties.
- Heat a lightly oiled skillet over medium heat and cook the patties for 3-4 minutes per side or until golden brown and cooked through.
- Serve with a side of sweet and sour sauce, shredded carrots and cucumbers, or steamed rice.

Tips and Variations:

You can use canned salmon for convenience, but be sure to drain and flake it before using.

Add other vegetables to the patties, such as chopped zucchini, carrots, or mushrooms.

For a gluten-free option, use almond flour or breadcrumbs instead of regular breadcrumbs.

Serve the patties with different sauces or dips, such as yoghurt sauce, avocado crema, or pesto.

Leftovers can be stored in an airtight container in the refrigerator for up to 3 days. Reheat gently in the oven or microwave.

Salmon and quinoa patties are a quick and easy meal that's packed with flavour and nutrition. Get creative with your ingredients and spices, and enjoy these delicious and versatile patties any time of the day!

Cauliflower and Chickpea Curry

Cauliflower and chickpea curry – a vegetarian delight that's bursting with flavour and warmth! Here are two flavorful variations to inspire your culinary journey:

Indian-Inspired Coconut Curry:
Ingredients:
- 1 tbsp vegetable oil
- 1 large onion, chopped
- 2 cloves garlic, minced
- 1 inch ginger, grated
- 1-2 tbsp curry powder (adjust to your spice preference)
- 1 tsp ground turmeric
- 1/2 tsp ground cumin
- 1/4 tsp chilli powder (optional)

- 1 can (14.5 oz) diced tomatoes
- 1 can (13.5 oz) coconut milk
- 1 head cauliflower, cut into florets
- 1 can (15 oz) chickpeas, drained and rinsed
- Salt and pepper to taste
- Fresh cilantro, chopped (for garnish)

Instructions:

- Heat oil in a large pot or Dutch oven over medium heat. Add onion and cook until softened about 5 minutes. Stir in garlic and ginger, and cook for 1 minute until fragrant.
- Add curry powder, turmeric, cumin, and chilli powder (if using). Cook for 30 seconds, stirring constantly to release the spices' aromas.
- Add tomatoes and coconut milk, and bring to a simmer. Stir in cauliflower and chickpeas, season with salt and pepper.
- Cover and simmer for 15-20 minutes or until cauliflower is tender. Adjust seasonings to taste.
- Garnish with chopped cilantro before serving.

Moroccan-Spiced Chickpea and Cauliflower Tagine:

Ingredients:

- 2 tbsp olive oil

- 1 onion, chopped
- 2 cloves garlic, minced
- 1 cinnamon stick
- 1 tsp coriander seeds
- 1/2 tsp ground turmeric
- 1/4 tsp paprika

Pinch of saffron (optional)

- 1 can (14.5 oz) diced tomatoes
- 1 cup vegetable broth
- 1 head cauliflower, cut into florets
- 1 can (15 oz) chickpeas, drained and rinsed
- 1/4 cup raisins (optional)
- 1/4 cup chopped almonds, toasted (for garnish)
- Chopped fresh parsley for garnish

Instructions:

Heat oil in a large pot or Dutch oven over medium heat. Add onion and cook until softened about 5 minutes. Stir in garlic, cinnamon stick, coriander seeds, turmeric, paprika, and saffron (if using). Cook for 1 minute until fragrant.

Add tomatoes and vegetable broth, and bring to a simmer. Stir in cauliflower and chickpeas, season with salt and pepper.

Cover and simmer for 20-25 minutes or until cauliflower is tender. Add raisins (if using) in the last 5 minutes of cooking.

Remove the cinnamon stick and discard. Serve garnished with toasted almonds and chopped parsley.

Tips and Variations:

For a richer curry, use full-fat coconut milk in the Indian version.

Add chopped bell peppers, spinach, or other vegetables to the curry for extra flavour and nutrients.

Replace cauliflower with broccoli or butternut squash for a different twist.

Serve the curry with rice, naan bread, or quinoa.

Top the Moroccan tagine with a dollop of plain yoghurt or harissa paste for a touch of coolness and spice.

No matter which variation you choose, cauliflower and chickpea curry is a satisfying and flavorful dish that's perfect for a cosy weeknight meal. So get creative, experiment with spices and ingredients, and enjoy this delicious and versatile vegetarian treasure!

Caprese Quinoa Bowl

The Caprese Quinoa Bowl is a delightful summery dish that combines the classic flavours of a Caprese salad with the nutritional and hearty goodness of quinoa. Here are two versions to tempt your taste buds:

Classic Caprese Quinoa Bowl:

Ingredients:

- 1 cup uncooked quinoa, rinsed
- 1 cup cherry tomatoes, halved
- 1/2 cup mozzarella pearls or cubed fresh mozzarella
- 1/4 cup chopped fresh basil
- 2 tablespoons olive oil
- 1 tablespoon balsamic vinegar
- Salt and pepper to taste

Instructions:

- Cook the quinoa according to package instructions. Fluff with a fork and let cool slightly.
- Divide the quinoa between two bowls. Top with cherry tomatoes, mozzarella, and basil.
- In a small bowl, whisk together olive oil, balsamic vinegar, salt, and pepper. Drizzle the dressing over the bowls.
- Serve immediately and enjoy!

Mediterranean Twist:

Ingredients:

- 1 cup uncooked quinoa, rinsed
- 1 cup chopped cucumber
- 1/2 cup crumbled feta cheese
- 1/4 cup chopped Kalamata olives

- 1/4 cup chopped red onion
- 2 tablespoons chopped fresh oregano
- 2 tablespoons red wine vinegar
- 1 tablespoon olive oil
- Salt and pepper to taste

Instructions:

- Cook the quinoa according to package instructions. Fluff with a fork and let cool slightly.
- Divide the quinoa between two bowls. Top with cucumber, feta cheese, olives, red onion, and oregano.
- In a small bowl, whisk together red wine vinegar, olive oil, salt, and pepper. Drizzle the dressing over the bowls.
- Serve immediately and enjoy!

Tips and Variations:

Drizzle the bowls with a touch of pesto for extra flavour.

Add grilled chicken or shrimp for a more substantial meal.

Toss in additional vegetables like roasted bell peppers, zucchini, or spinach.

Use brown rice or lentils instead of quinoa for a different twist.

Leftovers can be stored in an airtight container in the refrigerator for up to 3 days. Reheat gently in the microwave or oven.

The Caprese Quinoa Bowl is a versatile and satisfying dish that can be enjoyed for lunch, dinner, or even a light salad. Get creative with your ingredients and spices, and find your perfect flavour combination!

Turkey and Veggie Lettuce Wraps

Turkey and veggie lettuce wraps are a vibrant and delicious option for a light and healthy meal, perfect for summer picnics, quick dinners, or satisfying appetizers. Here are two variations to inspire your culinary creativity:

Asian-Inspired Lettuce Wraps:

Ingredients:

For the turkey:

- 1 pound ground turkey
- 1 tablespoon soy sauce
- 1 tablespoon oyster sauce (optional)
- 1 tablespoon rice vinegar
- 1 tablespoon sesame oil
- 1 tablespoon minced ginger
- 1 clove garlic, minced
- 1/2 teaspoon sriracha (optional)

- Salt and pepper to taste

For the wraps:

- 12 large butter lettuce leaves (or romaine or iceberg lettuce)
- 1 cup shredded carrots
- 1 cup chopped bell peppers (red, yellow, and orange)
- 1/2 cup sliced cucumber
- 1/4 cup chopped green onions
- 1/4 cup chopped fresh cilantro

Optional toppings: toasted peanuts, chopped peanuts, sesame seeds, sweet and sour sauce

Instructions:

- Combine the turkey, soy sauce, oyster sauce (if using), rice vinegar, sesame oil, ginger, garlic, sriracha (if using), salt, and pepper in a bowl. Mix well and set aside to marinate for at least 15 minutes.
- Heat a large skillet over medium heat. Add the marinated turkey and cook until browned and cooked through.
- While the turkey is cooking, wash and prepare the lettuce leaves. Shred the carrots and bell peppers, slice the cucumber, and chop the green onions and cilantro.

- Assemble the wraps by placing a spoonful of cooked turkey, some shredded carrots and bell peppers, sliced cucumber, chopped green onions, and cilantro on each lettuce leaf. Top with your desired toppings, and enjoy!

Mexican Fiesta Lettuce Wraps:

Ingredients:

For the turkey:

- 1 pound ground turkey
- 1 tablespoon taco seasoning
- 1 (15 oz) can diced tomatoes, undrained
- 1 (4 oz) can chopped green chiles, undrained
- 1/2 cup shredded cheddar cheese
- 1/4 cup chopped fresh cilantro
- Salt and pepper to taste

For the wraps:

- 12 large romaine lettuce leaves
- 1 cup black beans, rinsed and drained
- 1 cup chopped corn
- 1/2 cup chopped red onion
- 1/4 cup chopped fresh cilantro
- Optional toppings: avocado slices, sour cream, salsa, hot sauce

Instructions:

- Combine the ground turkey, taco seasoning, diced tomatoes, green chiles, cheddar cheese, cilantro, salt, and pepper in a bowl. Mix well and set aside.
- Heat a large skillet over medium heat. Add the turkey mixture and cook until browned and cooked through.
- While the turkey is cooking, wash and prepare the lettuce leaves. Rinse and drain the black beans. Chop the corn and red onion, and chop the cilantro.
- Assemble the wraps by placing a spoonful of cooked turkey, some black beans, corn, red onion, and cilantro on each lettuce leaf. Top with your desired toppings, and enjoy!

Tips and Variations:

Use ground chicken or tofu instead of ground turkey for different protein options.

Add other vegetables to the wraps, such as shredded cabbage, chopped lettuce, or sliced radishes.

Experiment with different sauces and toppings to find your perfect flavour combination.

Leftover fillings can be stored in an airtight container in the refrigerator for up to 3 days.

Turkey and veggie lettuce wraps are a delicious and versatile option for any meal. They're light, healthy, and can be easily customized to your liking. So get creative, have fun, and enjoy these flavorful wraps!

Sautéed Spinach with Garlic and Pine Nuts

sautéed spinach with garlic and pine nuts - a simple yet incredibly flavorful dish! It's a classic for a reason, offering a vibrant green side dish perfect for any occasion. Here are some tips and variations to get you started:

Basic Recipe:

Ingredients:

- 1 tablespoon olive oil
- 2 cloves garlic, minced
- 1/4 cup pine nuts
- 5 cups fresh spinach, washed and roughly chopped
- Salt and pepper to taste

Instructions:

- Heat the olive oil in a large skillet over medium heat. Add the garlic and cook until fragrant, about 30 seconds.
- Add the pine nuts and cook, stirring constantly, until lightly toasted, about 1-2 minutes.

- Add the spinach and cook, stirring frequently, until wilted and tender, about 2-3 minutes. Season with salt and pepper to taste.
- Serve immediately as a side dish or use as a base for other dishes like scrambled eggs or pasta.

Tips and Variations:

Spinach selection: Choose fresh, vibrant spinach with crisp leaves. Baby spinach works well for a more tender texture.

Olive oil: Opt for extra-virgin olive oil for the best flavour.

Garlic: Don't overcook the garlic, as it can burn and turn bitter.

Pine nuts: You can toast the pine nuts in a separate pan before adding them to the spinach for a deeper flavour.

Additional flavours: For a richer dish, add a squeeze of lemon juice, a pinch of red pepper flakes, or a spoonful of grated Parmesan cheese.

Protein boost: Add cooked shrimp, chicken, or tofu for a more substantial meal.

Pasta partner: Toss the sautéed spinach with cooked pasta, feta cheese, and a drizzle of olive oil for a quick and flavorful lunch or dinner.

Salad topping: Use the sautéed spinach as a warm topping for a mixed green salad.

Sautéed spinach with garlic and pine nuts is a quick, easy, and nutritious dish that can be enjoyed in countless ways. Get creative, experiment with different flavours and ingredients, and find your perfect version of this timeless classic!

Sweet Potato and Black Bean Quesadillas

Sweet potato and black bean quesadillas - a delightful fusion of sweet and savoury, perfect for a satisfying snack, lunch, or light dinner! Here are some recipe variations to inspire your culinary journey:

Classic Comfort:

Ingredients:

- 2 large sweet potatoes, peeled and thinly sliced
- 1 can (15 oz) black beans, drained and rinsed
- 1/2 cup shredded cheddar cheese
- 1/4 cup chopped red onion
- 1 tablespoon taco seasoning
- 1 tablespoon olive oil
- 4 large tortillas

Optional toppings: sour cream, salsa, guacamole

Instructions:

Heat olive oil in a large skillet over medium heat. Add sweet potatoes and cook, stirring occasionally, until softened and slightly browned, about 10-15 minutes.

Stir in black beans, taco seasoning, and red onion. Cook for another minute or two to heat through.

Place a tortilla on a plate or cutting board. Sprinkle with cheese and half of the sweet potato and black bean mixture. Fold the tortilla in half.

Heat a lightly oiled skillet over medium heat. Place the quesadilla in the pan and cook for 2-3 minutes per side or until golden brown and the cheese is melted.

Repeat with remaining tortillas and filling.

Serve with your desired toppings, and enjoy!

Southwestern Fusion:

Ingredients:

- 2 large sweet potatoes, peeled and diced
- 1 can (15 oz) black beans, drained and rinsed
- 1 cup frozen corn, thawed
- 1/2 cup chopped bell peppers (red, yellow, and orange)
- 1/4 cup chopped cilantro
- 1 tablespoon chilli powder
- 1 teaspoon cumin
- 1/2 teaspoon smoked paprika
- 1 tablespoon olive oil
- 4 large tortillas
- Optional toppings: avocado slices, cilantro lime crema, pico de gallo

Instructions:

- Heat olive oil in a large skillet over medium heat. Add sweet potatoes and cook, stirring occasionally, until softened and slightly browned, about 10-15 minutes.
- Add black beans, corn, bell peppers, and spices. Cook for another 3-4 minutes, until heated through.
- Stir in chopped cilantro just before serving.
- Assemble and cook quesadillas as per the classic recipe instructions.
- Top with your desired toppings, and enjoy!

Tips and Variations:

Use cooked sweet potato mash instead of diced potatoes for a quicker and softer filling.

Add other vegetables like mushrooms, zucchini, or spinach for extra flavour and nutrients.

For a vegan option, use vegan cheese or nutritional yeast for the topping.

You can bake the quesadillas in a preheated oven at 400°F (200°C) for 10-12 minutes, flipping halfway through cooking.

Leftovers can be stored in an airtight container in the refrigerator for up to 3 days. Reheat gently in a skillet or microwave.

Sweet potato and black bean quesadillas are a versatile and delicious dish that can be easily customized to your liking. So get creative, experiment with different flavours and ingredients, and enjoy this delightful fusion of sweet and savoury!

Mushroom and Spinach Stuffed Chicken Breast

Mushroom and spinach stuffed chicken breasts are a classic dish for a reason – they're packed with flavour, relatively easy to make, and offer endless variations to suit your taste buds. Here are a few recipe ideas to get you started:

Classic Creamy:

Ingredients:

- 4 boneless, skinless chicken breasts (around 7 oz each)
- 8 oz button mushrooms, chopped
- 1/2 cup chopped spinach
- 1 onion, chopped
- 2 cloves garlic, minced
- 1/4 cup shredded mozzarella cheese
- 1/4 cup ricotta cheese
- 1/4 cup milk
- 1 tablespoon olive oil

- 1/2 teaspoon dried thyme
- 1/4 teaspoon salt
- 1/4 teaspoon black pepper
- 1/4 cup chicken broth (optional)

Instructions:

Preheat oven to 375°F (190°C). Butterfly each chicken breast by carefully slicing it from the side, leaving it attached to the hinge. Open the chicken like a book.

In a skillet, heat olive oil and saute onions and garlic until softened. Add mushrooms and cook until lightly browned. Stir in spinach and cook until wilted.

Combine ricotta cheese, mozzarella cheese, milk, thyme, salt, and pepper. Mix with the mushroom and spinach mixture.

Stuff the chicken breasts with the filling, securing them closed with toothpicks if needed. Place in a baking dish.

Drizzle chicken with olive oil and season with salt and pepper. Bake for 20-25 minutes or until cooked through and juices run clear.

For a more decadent sauce, add chicken broth to the pan after draining excess fat and simmer for a few minutes before pouring over the cooked chicken.

Mediterranean Twist:

Ingredients:

Follow the same ingredients as the Classic Creamy recipe but replace herbs with:

- 1/2 teaspoon dried oregano
- 1/4 teaspoon dried rosemary
- Pinch of red pepper flakes (optional)

Add:

- 1/4 cup sun-dried tomatoes, chopped (oil-packed)
- 1/4 cup crumbled feta cheese (for topping)

Instructions:

- Follow the same instructions as the Classic Creamy recipe, incorporating the Mediterranean herb substitutions and adding sun-dried tomatoes to the stuffing.
- Top with crumbled feta cheese before serving.

Tips and Variations:

Use other mushrooms like chanterelles or portobellos for a richer flavour.

Add crumbled cooked bacon or sausage to the stuffing for a heartier dish.

Stuff the chicken breasts with a mixture of spinach and other greens like kale or arugula.

Use different cheeses like goat cheese, blue cheese, or Gruyere for a different flavour profile.

Wrap the chicken breasts in prosciutto or bacon before baking for an extra burst of savoury goodness.

Serve with mashed potatoes, rice, or roasted vegetables for a complete meal.

No matter which variation you choose, mushroom and spinach stuffed chicken breasts are sure to be a crowd-pleaser. So get creative, experiment with different flavours and ingredients, and enjoy this delicious and versatile dish!

Quinoa and Vegetable Stir-Fry

Quinoa and vegetable stir-fry is a fantastically versatile and healthy dish, perfect for any occasion. Here are some recipe ideas to inspire your culinary journey:

Classic Comfort:

Ingredients:

- 1 cup uncooked quinoa, cooked and fluffed
- 1 tablespoon olive oil
- 1 onion, chopped
- 1 bell pepper (red, yellow, or orange), chopped
- 1 carrot, chopped
- 1 cup broccoli florets
- 1/2 cup peas

- 2 cloves garlic, minced
- 1/4 cup soy sauce
- 1 tablespoon sesame oil
- 1 tablespoon rice vinegar
- 1 teaspoon sriracha (optional)
- Salt and pepper to taste

Instructions:

Heat olive oil in a large wok or skillet over medium heat. Add onion and cook until softened about 5 minutes.

Add bell pepper, carrot, and broccoli, and cook for another 5 minutes or until slightly tender. Stir in peas.

Add garlic and cook for 30 seconds until fragrant.

In a small bowl, whisk together soy sauce, sesame oil, rice vinegar, and sriracha (if using). Add to the pan and stir-fry for 1 minute.

Add cooked quinoa and cook for another minute or two until heated through. Season with salt and pepper to taste.

Serve immediately with optional toppings like sliced green onions, toasted sesame seeds, or chopped peanuts.

Asian Fusion:

Ingredients:

Follow the same ingredients as the Classic Comfort recipe but replace vegetables with:

- 1 cup snow peas

- 1 cup chopped bok choy
- 1/2 cup sliced water chestnuts
- 1/4 cup shredded red cabbage

Add:

- 1 teaspoon grated ginger
- 1/2 teaspoon crushed red pepper flakes (optional)
- 1 tablespoon oyster sauce (optional)

Instructions:

- Follow the same instructions as the Classic Comfort recipe, incorporating the Asian fusion substitutions and adding ginger and red pepper flakes (if using) with the garlic.
- Use the oyster sauce in place of some of the soy sauce for a deeper umami flavour.

Tips and Variations:

Use any vegetables you like! Add zucchini, corn, mushrooms, or green beans for additional flavour and texture.

Replace quinoa with brown rice or another whole grain for a different twist.

Make it vegan by using vegetable broth instead of chicken broth and skipping the optional oyster sauce.

Add cooked protein like chicken, shrimp, or tofu for a more substantial meal.

Top with a fried egg for a satisfying protein boost.

Drizzle with sweet and sour sauce, peanut sauce, or sriracha for different flavour profiles.

No matter which variation you choose, quinoa and vegetable stir-fry is sure to be a healthy and delicious meal. So get creative, experiment with different flavours and ingredients, and enjoy this versatile dish!

Lemon Garlic Roasted Broccoli

Lemon garlic roasted broccoli is a simple yet incredibly flavorful side dish that packs a punch of vitamins and antioxidants. Here are two variations to inspire your culinary journey:

Classic Comfort:

Ingredients:

- 1 head broccoli, cut into florets
- 2 tablespoons olive oil
- 1 tablespoon lemon juice
- 2 cloves garlic, minced
- 1/2 teaspoon salt
- 1/4 teaspoon black pepper

Optional toppings: Parmesan cheese, red pepper flakes, chopped fresh parsley

Instructions:

- Preheat oven to 425°F (220°C).
- Toss broccoli florets with olive oil, lemon juice, garlic, salt, and pepper in a large bowl.
- Spread the broccoli on a baking sheet in a single layer.
- Roast for 15-20 minutes or until tender and slightly browned.
- Serve immediately with your desired toppings, and enjoy!

Mediterranean Twist:

Ingredients:

Follow the same ingredients as the Classic Comfort recipe but add:

- 1/2 teaspoon dried oregano
- Pinch of red pepper flakes (optional)
- Kalamata olives, sliced (optional)
- Feta cheese, crumbled (optional)

Instructions:

- Follow the same instructions as the Classic Comfort recipe, incorporating the Mediterranean herb and spice additions.
- Top with sliced Kalamata olives and crumbled feta cheese before serving (optional).

Tips and Variations:

For a crispier texture, preheat the baking sheet before adding the broccoli.

Add other vegetables like Brussels sprouts, red onion, or bell peppers for a rainbow of flavours.

For a smoky flavour, add a teaspoon of smoked paprika to the seasoning mix.

Sprinkle with Parmesan cheese or nutritional yeast for a vegan cheese-like flavour.

Drizzle with balsamic glaze or sriracha for a touch of sweetness or heat.

Leftovers can be stored in an airtight container in the refrigerator for up to 3 days. Reheat gently in the oven or microwave.

Lemon garlic roasted broccoli is a versatile and delicious side dish that can be enjoyed with meat, fish, pasta, or as a snack on its own. Get creative, experiment with different flavours and ingredients, and enjoy this healthy and flavorful dish!

Vegetarian Tacos with Avocado Cream

Vegetarian tacos are a vibrant and delicious way to enjoy a plant-based meal, and adding avocado cream elevates them to a whole new level! Here are two enticing variations to tempt your taste buds:

Roasted Veggie Bliss:

Ingredients:

For the roasted veggies:

- 1 zucchini, diced
- 1 bell pepper (red, yellow, or orange), diced
- 1 red onion, diced
- 1 tablespoon olive oil
- 1/2 teaspoon dried oregano
- 1/4 teaspoon smoked paprika
- Salt and pepper to taste

For the tacos:

- 4 corn tortillas
- 1 can (15 oz) black beans, drained and rinsed
- 1 cup chopped romaine lettuce
- 1/2 cup sliced cherry tomatoes
- 1/4 cup crumbled queso fresco (optional)
- For the avocado cream:
- 1 ripe avocado
- 1/4 cup lime juice
- 1/4 cup chopped cilantro
- 1 clove garlic, minced
- Pinch of salt and pepper

Instructions:

- Preheat oven to 425°F (220°C). Toss the diced vegetables with olive oil, oregano, paprika, salt, and pepper. Spread on a baking sheet and roast for 15-20 minutes or until tender and slightly browned.

- While veggies are roasting, prepare the avocado cream. Blend all ingredients in a food processor or blender until smooth and creamy.
- Warm the tortillas according to package instructions.
- Fill each tortilla with black beans, roasted veggies, romaine lettuce, and cherry tomatoes.
- Drizzle with a generous dollop of avocado cream and top with queso fresco (optional). Enjoy!

Spicy Bean and Sweet Potato Fiesta:

Ingredients:

For the bean filling:

- 1 can (15 oz) black beans, drained and rinsed
- 1 can (15 oz) pinto beans, drained and rinsed
- 1 small sweet potato, peeled and diced
- 1 onion, chopped
- 1 jalapeno, seeded and minced (adjust for desired spice level)
- 1 tablespoon olive oil
- 1 tablespoon chilli powder
- 1 teaspoon cumin
- 1/2 teaspoon smoked paprika

- Salt and pepper to taste

For the tacos:

- 4 corn tortillas
- 1 cup chopped romaine lettuce
- 1/2 cup chopped red onion
- 1/4 cup sliced avocado
- 1/4 cup chopped fresh cilantro
- Lime wedges
- For the avocado cream (optional):
- Same recipe as above

Instructions:

- Heat olive oil in a large skillet over medium heat. Add onion and jalapeno and cook until softened about 5 minutes.
- Add spices and cook for 30 seconds until fragrant.
- Add sweet potato and cook for 5 minutes or until softened.
- Stir in black beans, pinto beans, and a splash of water. Bring to a simmer and cook for 5 minutes, allowing flavours to meld. Season with salt and pepper to taste.
- Warm the tortillas according to package instructions.
- Fill each tortilla with bean mixture, romaine lettuce, red onion, avocado, and cilantro.

- Drizzle with lime juice and serve with avocado cream (optional).

Tips and Variations:

Use other vegetables like mushrooms, zucchini, or corn for the roasted veggie taco variation.

Add cooked tofu, tempeh, or jackfruit for a protein boost.

Top the spicy bean and sweet potato tacos with shredded cheese, sour cream, or salsa.

Play with different herbs and spices like chipotle chili powder, smoked paprika, or coriander in the fillings.

Serve the tacos with other toppings like pickled onions, radishes, or jicama slaw.

For a gluten-free option, use corn tortillas or lettuce wraps.

Vegetarian tacos with avocado cream are a versatile and delicious dish that can be easily customized to your liking. Get creative, experiment with different flavours and ingredients, and enjoy this vibrant and flavorful fiesta!

CONCLUSION

The Dietary Approaches to Stop Hypertension, commonly known as the DASH diet, has emerged as a holistic and effective approach to promoting heart health and overall well-being. With a primary focus on reducing blood pressure, the DASH diet has garnered widespread recognition for its potential to prevent and manage cardiovascular diseases. In this comprehensive conclusion, we will delve into the key principles of the DASH diet, its proven health benefits, potential challenges, and the broader implications for public health.

The DASH diet places a strong emphasis on consuming a well-balanced and nutrient-rich diet that is low in sodium. Central to its principles is the promotion of fruits, vegetables, whole grains, lean proteins, and dairy products while minimizing the intake of saturated fats, cholesterol, and added sugars. This balanced approach aligns with established nutritional guidelines and is supported by a wealth of scientific evidence.

One of the undeniable strengths of the DASH diet is its effectiveness in lowering blood pressure. Numerous studies have demonstrated a consistent reduction in both systolic and diastolic blood pressure among individuals following the DASH eating plan. This reduction is especially noteworthy given the prevalence of hypertension and its association with an increased risk of heart disease, stroke, and other cardiovascular complications.

Beyond its impact on blood pressure, the DASH diet has been linked to a range of other health benefits. Its emphasis on whole foods rich in vitamins, minerals, and antioxidants contributes to improved overall cardiovascular health. The diet's positive effects extend to cholesterol levels, with reductions in LDL cholesterol observed in various studies. Additionally, the DASH diet has been associated with better insulin sensitivity, making it a valuable tool in the prevention and management of type 2 diabetes.

The adaptability of the DASH diet further enhances its appeal. Whether individuals are seeking to control hypertension, manage weight, or promote general well-being, the DASH principles can be tailored to meet diverse health goals. This flexibility is underscored by the availability of different versions of the DASH diet, including those accommodating specific dietary preferences such as vegetarian or vegan lifestyles.

Despite the numerous advantages of the DASH diet, challenges exist in its widespread adoption. Barriers may include cultural preferences, economic constraints, and the omnipresence of processed and convenience foods that often contain high levels of sodium and unhealthy fats. Addressing these challenges requires a multi-faceted approach that combines education, policy changes, and increased accessibility to affordable, healthy food options.

The impact of the DASH diet extends beyond individual health to broader public health implications. As societies grapple with rising rates of obesity, cardiovascular diseases, and associated healthcare costs, promoting dietary patterns like the DASH diet becomes imperative. Public health campaigns and interventions should prioritize raising awareness about the benefits of the DASH diet, providing practical resources, and fostering environments conducive to healthy eating.

Furthermore, the DASH diet aligns with sustainable and environmentally conscious food choices. By promoting the consumption of plant-based foods, whole grains, and lean proteins, the DASH diet supports a more ecologically responsible approach to nutrition. As global concerns about climate change and resource depletion intensify, the environmental impact of dietary choices should be a crucial consideration in public health recommendations.

In conclusion, the DASH diet stands as a beacon of evidence-based nutrition, offering a roadmap to improved cardiovascular health and overall well-being. Its emphasis on a balanced and nutrient-dense diet, coupled with proven effectiveness in lowering blood pressure and promoting various health benefits, positions it as a valuable tool in the prevention and management of chronic diseases. As we navigate the complex landscape of modern dietary patterns and their impact on health, the DASH diet serves as a compelling model for individuals, healthcare professionals, and policymakers alike. Embracing the principles of the DASH diet has the potential to not only transform individual lives but also contribute to a healthier and more resilient society.